Devices in Cardiac Critical Care

Notice

Medicine is an ever-changing science. As new research and clinical experience broaden our knowledge, changes in treatment and drug therapy are required. The authors and the publisher of this work have checked with sources believed to be reliable in their efforts to provide information that is complete and generally in accord with the standards accepted at the time of publication. However, in view of the possibility of human error or changes in medical sciences, neither the authors nor the publisher nor any other party who has been involved in the preparation or publication of this work warrants that the information contained herein is in every respect accurate or complete, and they disclaim all responsibility for any errors or omissions or for the results obtained from use of the information contained in this work. Readers are encouraged to confirm the information contained herein with other sources. For example and in particular, readers are advised to check the product information sheet included in the package of each drug they plan to administer to be certain that the information contained in this work is accurate and that changes have not been made in the recommended dose or in the contraindications for administration. This recommendation is of particular importance in connection with new or infrequently used drugs.

Devices in Cardiac Critical Care

Editors

Samin K. Sharma, MD
Professor of Cardiology
Mount Sinai Hospital
New York, New York

Timothy J. Vittorio, MS, MD
Department of Cardiology
BronxCare Hospital Center
Bronx, New York

Muhammad Saad, MD
Department of Advanced Heart Failure and Transplant
Mount Sinai Hospital
New York, New York

1 2 3 4 5 6 7 8 9   LCR   29 28 27 26 25 24

ISBN 978-1-265-20961-2
MHID 1-265-20961-8

This book was set in Minion Pro by KnowledgeWorks Global Ltd.
The editors were Timothy Y. Hiscock and Kim J. Davis.
The production supervisor was Richard Ruzycka.
Project management was provided by Nitesh Sharma of KnowledgeWorks Global Ltd.
The cover designer was W2 Design.

This book is printed on acid-free paper.

Library of Congress Cataloging-in-Publication Data

Names: Sharma, Samin K., editor. | Saad, Muhammad, MD, editor. | Vittorio, Timothy J, editor.
Title: Devices in cardiac critical care / editors, Samin Sharma, Muhammad Saad, Timothy J. Vittorio.
Description: New York : McGraw Hill, [2024] | Includes bibliographical references and index. | Summary: "This book will serve as an effective teaching tool regarding the appropriateness and utilization of cardiac devices in the cardiac critical care unit"—Provided by publisher.
Identifiers: LCCN 2023042877 (print) | LCCN 2023042878 (ebook) | ISBN 9781265209612 (paperback ; alk. paper) | ISBN 9781265210830 (ebook)
Subjects: MESH: Cardiovascular Diseases—therapy | Equipment and Supplies | Critical Care | Case Reports
Classification: LCC RC669 (print) | LCC RC669 (ebook) | NLM WG 26 | DDC 616.1/028—dc23/eng/20231208
LC record available at https://lccn.loc.gov/2023042877
LC ebook record available at https://lccn.loc.gov/2023042878

McGraw Hill books are available at special quantity discounts to use as premiums and sales promotions or for use in corporate training programs. To contact a representative, please visit the Contact Us pages at www.mhprofessional.com.

I dedicate this book to my father, trainees, and patients for their constant inspiration and support.

—Samin K. Sharma

I dedicate this book to my family for their constant support, encouragement, patience, and love.
Thank you as well to my mentors, teachers, and colleagues for shaping my medical education
and making me the physician I am today. Most of all,
I dedicate this book to the patients who have entrusted me with their care.

—Timothy J. Vittorio

To my parents (Saeeda Azhar and Azhar Hussain), for all the care and love you have provided to us.
To my wife (Wajiha Saad) and daughters (Zariyah Saad, Fabiha Saad, and Fatima Saad)
for creating peaceful environment for me to prosper.
To all my siblings (Fareeha, Ashar, and Anas) for always supporting me. Finally, to all my mentors,
colleagues, and juniors for a great inspiration to me, thank you all.

—Muhammad Saad

Contents

Contributors

Fareeha Alavi
Attending
University of Maryland Charles Regional Hospital
La Plata, Maryland

Nisha Ali, MD
Department of Cardiology
Mount Sinai Morningside—BronxCare Health System
New York, New York

Sai Vishnuvardhan Allu, MD
Resident Physician
Department of Internal Medicine
BronxCare Hospital
Bronx, New York

Shoaib Ashraf, MD
Cardiology Fellow PGY4
Mount Sinai Morningside
New York, New York

Iqra Bhatti
Medical Student
American University of the Caribbean
St. Louis, Missouri

Angel de la Cruz, MD
Cardiology Fellow
Mount Sinai Morningside
New York, New York

Arundhati Dileep, MD
Cardiology Fellow
Mount Sinai Morningside
New York, New York

Umesh K. Gidwani, MD, MS, FCCM, FACC, FCCP
Chief, Cardiac Critical Care
Zena and Michael A. Wiener Cardiovascular Institute
Director, Cardiac ICU, Mount Sinai Hospital
Institute for Critical Care Medicine
Professor of Medicine
Icahn School of Medicine at Mount Sinai
New York, New York

Muhammad T. Hassan
Medical Student
Department of Cardiology
BronxCare Hospital Center
Bronx, New York

Vibha Hayagreev, MD
Resident
BronxCare Hospital Center
Bronx, New York

Charbel Ishak, MD
Attending Interventional Radiology
BronxCare Hospital
Bronx, New York

Preeti Jadhav, MD
Interventional Cardiology Faculty
Associate Program Director
BronxCare Hospital Systems—Mount Sinai Morningside
  Cardiovascular Disease Fellowship
Icahn School of Medicine at Mount Sinai
New York, New York

Wajiha Jahangir, MD
Department of Internal Medicine
BronxCare Hospital
Bronx, New York

Maheen A. Khan
Medical Student
Department of Cardiology
BronxCare Hospital Center
Bronx, New York

Sneha Khannal
Resident
BronxCare Hospital Center
Bronx, New York

Sarthak Kulshreshtha, MD
UIC College of Medicine Residency Program
Rockford, Illinois

Jeirym Miranda, MD
Department of Advanced Cardiovascular Imaging
Montefiore Hospital Center
Bronx, New York

Muhammad Khuram Nouman, MD
Resident
BronxCare Hospital Center
Bronx, New York

Emamuzo Obaro Otobo, MD
Cardiology Fellow
Mount Sinai Morningside
New York, New York

Neelanjana Pandey, MD
PGY-4 Chief Resident
Department of Internal Medicine
BronxCare Health System
Affiliated to Icahn School of Medicine
Bronx, New York

Muhammad Saad, MD
Department of Advance Heart Failure and Transplant
Mount Sinai Hospital
New York, New York

Gregory Serrao, MD
Interventional Cardiology
Mount Sinai Hospital
New York, New York

Niel Shah, MD
Attending
Jefferson Einstein Hospital
Philadelphia, Pennsylvania

Tamir D. Vittorio
SUNY Binghamton Harpur College of Arts and Sciences
Binghamton, New York

Timothy J. Vittorio, MS, MD
Department of Cardiology
BronxCare Hospital Center
Bronx, New York

Preface

The first edition of our textbook *Devices in Cardiac Critical Care* was devised as a practical and unique means to assist physicians-in-training including internal medicine residents, cardiology fellows, nurse practitioners, physician assistants, and medical students who rotate on a busy tertiary cardiac critical care unit. We constructed the text to be as user-friendly as possible by utilizing a personal conversation style of writing.

This textbook is essentially a user's manual to assist the medical practitioner in making adequate clinical judgment. The book is divided into chapters based on genuine clinical cases with a proposed approach for each case.

To help orient and to prevent excessive details to the reader, we included several key points in each case complementing and highlighting the major points throughout the clinical content with the intention of allowing an easier and faster review.

It is our goal that this book serves as an effective teaching tool regarding the appropriateness and utilization of cardiac devices in the cardiac critical care unit.

We hope that you enjoy this book and find it useful.

Samin K. Sharma, MD
Timothy J. Vittorio, MD
Muhammad Saad, MD

Devices in Cardiac Critical Care

Resuscitation Devices

CHAPTER 1

• *Neelanjana Pandey, MD; Iqra Bhatti, MD; Timothy J. Vittorio, MD*

■ CASE PRESENTATION

History of present illness: A 55-year-old man was at his office desk when his coworker noticed him frothing from the mouth and subsequently losing consciousness. The coworker activated 911 and immediately began cardiopulmonary resuscitation (CPR). When the emergency medical service (EMS) arrived, the initial rhythm demonstrated ventricular fibrillation (VF). Advanced cardiac life support (ACLS) was implemented, and return of spontaneous circulation (ROSC) was achieved in 10 minutes. However, there were repeated episodes of VF requiring multiple defibrillation attempts along with repeated episodes of CPR, and the patient remained unresponsive. While en route to the nearest hospital, he was orally intubated and a 12-lead electrocardiogram (ECG) was performed, revealing ST-segment elevations in the anterior precordial leads.

Past medical history: Hypertension (HTN), diabetes mellitus type 2 (DMT2).

Past surgical history: No surgeries in the past.

Family history: Father with a history of HTN. Mother with a history of DMT2.

Social history: Current active smoker: 1 pack per day for 20 years, no illicit drug use.

Allergies: No known drug allergies.

Home medications: Amlodipine, metformin, rosuvastatin.

Physical examination:

  Blood pressure: 80/50 mmHg

  Heart rate: 100 bpm

  Respiratory rate: 24 rpm

  Temperature: 97.4°F

  SpO$_2$: 98% on mechanical ventilation

  GA: Orally intubated, sedated

  HEENT: Normocephalic, atraumatic

  Lungs: Bilateral normal vesicular breath sounds, no wheezes or crackles

  Heart: S$_1$ and S$_2$ normal in intensity; no audible murmurs, rubs, or gallops

  Abdomen: Soft, nontender, nondistended

  Extremities: No pedal edema

  Neurologic: Unresponsive

The patient also required multiple episodes of defibrillation in the emergency department. Subsequently, he was transferred to the cardiac catheterization laboratory. Emergency medical personnel initiated therapeutic hypothermia (TH) for him by placing water blankets, cooling caps, and a cooling catheter that remained in place during the cardiac catheterization procedure. A selective coronary arteriogram revealed complete occlusion of the proximal left anterior descending (LAD) coronary artery, which was revascularized using a drug-eluting stent (DES). On arrival to the cardiac intensive care unit (CICU), TH was continued for about 24 hours, and the patient was slowly rewarmed. Initially, he remained comatose. By day 5, he was awake, alert, and interactive and was ultimately discharged home.

KEY POINTS

- Cardiac arrest is often a sudden and catastrophic event that needs prompt attention to hypoxia, hypovolemia, hypothermia, pneumothorax, myocardial infraction, tamponade, and pulmonary embolism.
- Early resuscitation with airway management, early CPR, defibrillation, and ACLS support are required to improve survival.

COMPONENTS OF RESUSCITATION DEVICES (FIGURE 1-1)

Cardiopulmonary arrest consists of sudden cessation of the circulatory system leading to global ischemia. Out-of-hospital arrest occurs at home in the majority of the cases, with middle-aged men as the main victims. Early initiation of resuscitation efforts by trained personnel has shown outcome benefits. Resuscitation consists of the following components.

Airway Devices

Bag Valve Mask

Introduction The bag valve mask (BVM) was first developed in 1965 and is used to provide positive-pressure ventilation to individuals who are not breathing or are having difficulty breathing. It is frequently used in hospitals and other civilian settings.

Indications BVMs can maintain airway patency until definite airway control is established. It is especially useful in providing temporary respiratory support in emergency situations such as respiratory failure, impending respiratory arrest, and apnea.

Contraindications There is no medical contraindication to giving ventilation support except for a do-not-resuscitate (DNR) order in place.

Mechanism of Working A BVM consists of a resuscitator bag with a non-rebreathing valve mechanism and a soft mask that conforms to the tissue of the face and gets connected to the oxygen supply. (See Figure 1-2.)

The mask needs to fit securely against the face to avoid leaking; the bag is then manually compressed and the patient is ventilated through the nose and mouth.

Resuscitator bags can be used with either oropharyngeal or nasopharyngeal airways or can be used with artificial airways such as endotracheal tubes. BVM can be applied using 1 or 2 people; a tight seal is created more effectively with 2 hands on the mask.

A positive end-expiratory pressure (PEEP) valve is sometimes used to improve oxygenation as it will improve alveolar recruitment and therefore oxygenation.

Complications If BVM ventilation is used for a long time and improperly, it can introduce air into the stomach

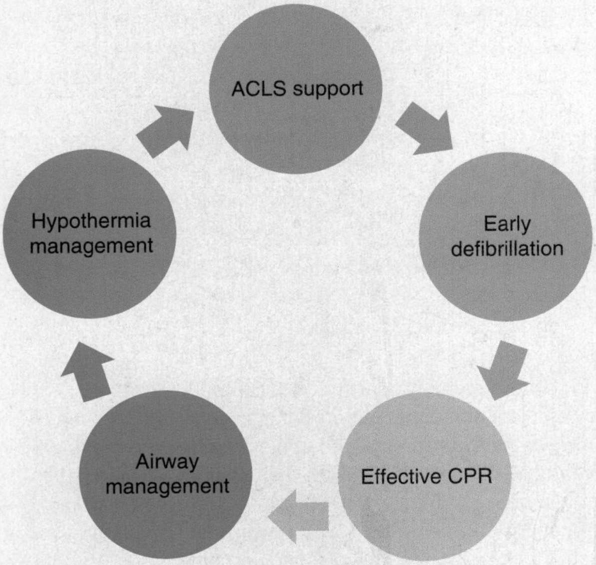

FIGURE 1-1. Components of resuscitation devices.

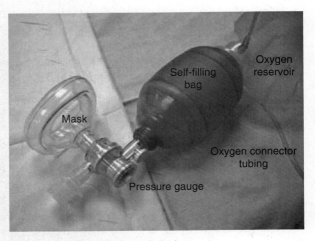

FIGURE 1-2. Bag valve mask device.

and cause gastric distention. Other complications include hyperventilation, vomiting, and aspiration.

Trouble Shooting Some of the factors to help troubleshoot if ventilation becomes difficult include the following. Presence of facial hair or facial trauma can create an inadequate mask seal. Increased soft tissue mass in people with obesity may also cause obstruction, more often when the patient is obtunded. The absence of teeth may also interfere with adequate ventilation, and in such cases, a supraglottic airway might be helpful.

Laryngeal Mask Airway (Figure 1-3)
Introduction A laryngeal mask airway (LMA) is the most commonly used supraglottic airway for advanced airway management. When it was introduced in the 1980s, its use was primarily restricted to the operating room (OR) and intensive care unit (ICU); however, it is now widely used as an alternative to BVM in the emergency room and field settings.

Indications LMAs are indicated primarily as a bridge to intubation in patients with sudden cardiac arrest (SCA) or to provide temporary ventilation in a patient with a failed airway. It is an excellent alternative to BVM as the chances of gastric distention and risk of aspiration are reduced.

Contraindications LMAs should not be used in conscious or awake patients, as this might stimulate the gag reflex. Absolute contraindications include underlying pharyngeal pathology, poor lung compliance, massive facial trauma, and airway obstruction below the larynx.

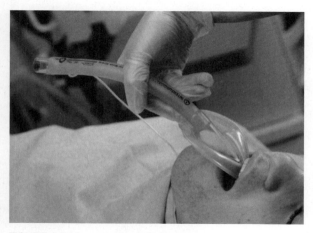

FIGURE 1-3. Laryngeal mask airway.

Mechanism of Action LMAs have different forms depending on the manufacturer. However, the basic structure remains the same, consisting of a tube connected to an inflatable cuff that covers the supraglottic area.

This can facilitate an open airway and allow for spontaneous or positive-pressure ventilation (PPV). It is inserted into the lower oropharynx to prevent airway obstruction by soft tissues and create effective ventilation.

These devices seal the laryngeal inlet instead of the face-mask (FM) interface; hence, vomiting and aspiration are the most common side effects, especially in patients with an intact gag reflex.

LMA is inserted by pressing the deflated mask against the hard palate and rotating it past the base of the tongue until the mask reaches the hypopharynx.

Newer devices can provide higher seal pressures and allow for easier intubation; they also have a gastric access port to aspirate gastric contents and incorporate a bite block.

Complications Prolonged use and overinflation of the device can compress the tongue, leading to tongue edema. Other complications from the procedure include vomiting, coughing, laryngospasm, lingual artery compression, and transient hypoglossal nerve paralysis.

Additionally, rare cases of pneumomediastinum and subcutaneous emphysema have also been reported.

Trouble Shooting Some of the factors to help troubleshoot if ventilation becomes difficult include difficult anatomy and restricted mouth opening, which will not allow passage of the device.

Upper or lower airway obstruction due to a foreign body and tumor may cause difficulty in passing the LMA. Obesity predisposes to an inadequate positioning of the device, leading to leaks.

Short thyromental distance leads to difficult positioning of the tongue and hence difficulty in placing extraglottic devices such as LMAs.

Endotracheal Tube
Introduction An endotracheal tube (ETT) is the most definitive method to secure a compromised airway in patients who need prolonged mechanical ventilation.

Laryngoscopy involves visualization of vocal cords either directly or assisted by video. An ETT can be placed directly into the trachea as well as via cricothyrotomy.

Indication ETT is indicated in clinical conditions such as poor oxygenation, poor ventilation, altered mental status, hypercarbia, and questionable airway patency.

A Glasgow coma scale score of 8 or lower is also an indication to intubate the patient.

Contraindications Severe facial trauma is a relative contraindication to oropharyngeal intubation. Because ETT involves spine manipulation, in patients with an underlying spine injury or immobility, intubation might be risky.

There is no absolute contraindication to intubation. Definitive airway placement is based on clinical judgment and the patient's condition.

Mechanism of Action Preparation for ETT starts with optimizing the position of the patient and setting up the preoxygenation equipment.

ETT is inserted into the trachea, which is part of the lower airway, connecting the upper airway (oral cavity and pharynx) to the lungs. It has cartilaginous rings anteriorly and is soft and membranous posteriorly. These features differentiate it from the esophagus.

ETT is inserted using a stylet via direct laryngoscopy, and a cuff is inflated with air through a syringe connected to the side port.

Generally, a size 7 is used for women and 8 for men; however, size may vary depending on the patient's height. The balloon cuffs prevent air leakage and minimize the chances of aspiration. They also permit suctioning of the lower respiratory tract. Rapid sequence intubation is the most commonly used method; it involves a sedative and a paralytic agent, is quick in onset, and has a short duration of action.

Complications The most feared complication of intubation is hypoxemia due to multiple attempts in placing the tube as a result of difficult intubation or a misplaced tube.

To avoid this, ETT placement needs to be immediately confirmed. Laryngoscopy may be used in patients with anticipated difficult airways.

Laryngoscopy can cause vagal stimulation, leading to bradycardia. Additionally, sedative medications have the potential for causing hypotension, especially in critically ill patients, which can lead to hemodynamic compromise and SCA.

Other complications include esophageal intubation, frank aspiration, trauma to the teeth, and laceration of the oropharynx.

Trouble Shooting Evaluation of external anatomy can help predict a difficult airway, such as in patients with restricted cervical motion or facial and neck trauma.

In anticipated difficult intubation, it is preferred to use video-assisted laryngoscopy, which has a curved blade.

If the first attempt to intubate is unsuccessful, then a tracheal tube introducer called a bougie can be used, which is a flexible device introduced to allow for identification of the cartilaginous part of the airway.

ETT position is confirmed with the help of end-tidal carbon dioxide ($EtCO_2$) monitoring. In extratracheal intubation, such as esophageal or hypopharyngeal intubation, $EtCO_2$ will record 0 mmHg. Postintubation chest radiography can confirm the location of the ETT, which should be 2 to 4 cm proximal to the carina.

Automated External Defibrillation (Figure 1-4)

A defibrillator is a device that sends an electrical impulse or shock to the heart to restore normal rhythm. It can be used to correct or prevent an arrhythmia and can prevent sudden cardiac death.

There are 2 types of external defibrillators:

- Public access automated external defibrillation (AED): Used by public/layman in public area and requires minimal training.
- Professional access AED: Used by medical personnel and requires training.

Time to defibrillation is the most important determinant of survival for VF and pulseless ventricular tachycardia (VT) with an increase in mortality of 7% to 10% for every 1-minute delay in defibrillation. Layman use of AED is associated with improved neurologic outcomes.

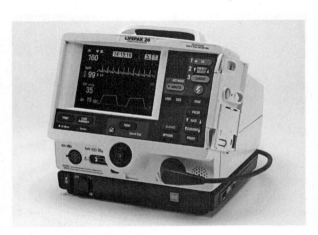

FIGURE 1-4. Defibrillator device.

Indication and Contraindications Immediate electrical shock is required for the treatment of VF and pulseless VT to achieve ROSC.

Contraindications include a DNR order and if the patient is conscious and has a palpable pulse.

Mechanism of Work AED is a portable device that will analyze the heart's rhythm in people experiencing cardiac arrest. It is usually found in public places, also known as public access AEDs and can be used by bystanders in case of an emergency. Before activating AED, expert help should be called. Professional AEDs are used by first responders.

Each AED device comes with pads or sensors, also called electrodes, with instructions on how to place them on the person's chest. The device also comes with 2 buttons: analyze and shock. The analyze button will analyze the rhythm to find out if shock is needed. Some AEDs have a variable intensity of shock starting from 90 J and increasing to 120, 150, and up to 300 J.

Complications Low-energy shocks are not painful but feel like fluttering in the chest. High-energy shocks can be strong or painful.

Cardiac contusion, rhabdomyolysis from multiple shocks, and skin burn can occur.

Trouble Shooting The AED provides prompts, such as if pads are not detected (AED should be repositioned) or if the patient has hairy skin (that area can be shaved).

If the skin is wet, pads will not attach, leading to inadequate energy delivery. All movements and chest compressions should be stopped before defibrillation.

Hypothermia Devices

Introduction

Therapeutic hypothermia (TH) improves survival rates and brain function in post-SCA patients. The temperature of the body is lowered to 89°F to 93°F for 24 hours.

TH is divided into 4 stages: initiation, maintenance, rewarming, and return to normothermia. It should be initiated as soon as possible after achieving ROSC with a target temperature range of 32°C to 34°C. There is a 20% increase in mortality for every hour of delay in the initiation of TH.

Three methods include transnasal evaporative cooling, water blankets, and cooling caps. The most commonly used method is cooling catheters (Figure 1-5).

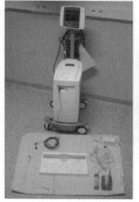
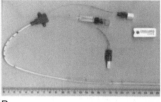

B

A

FIGURE 1-5. Cooling catheter equipment.

Cooling catheters allow precise temperature management using a central venous catheter, through which cool or warm saline circulates in a closed loop, cooling or warming a patient as venous blood passes over the balloons without infusing saline into the patient.

Indications

As per current American Heart Association (AHA) guidelines, TH is a Class I recommendation if the arrest is from VT or VF and a Class IIb recommendation for SCA from other nonshockable rhythms. (See Table 1-1.)

■ TABLE 1-1. Recommendations for Targeted Temperature Management (TTM) Indications		
Recommendations for Indications TTM		
COR	**LOE**	**Recommendations**
1	B-R	1. We recommend TTM for adults who do not follow commands after ROSC from OHCA with any initial rhythm.
1	B-R	2. We recommend TTM for adults who do not follow commands after ROSC from IHCA with initial nonshockable rhythm.
1	B-NR	3. We recommend TTM for adults who do not follow commands after ROSC from IHCA with initial nonshockable rhythm.

Abbreviations: COR, class of recommendation; IHCA, in-hospital cardiac arrest; LOE, level of evidence; OHCA, out-of-hospital cardiac arrest.

Contraindications

TH is contraindicated in patients with intracranial hemorrhage (ICH), hypotension requiring multiple intravenous vasopressors, severe sepsis, pregnancy, and severe hemorrhage.

Complications

Shivering is natural and the most common reaction to cooling. It should be recognized early and treated aggressively as it will increase the metabolic rate and prevent one from achieving the target temperature.

Shivering can be avoided by wrapping the body with warm blankets, and magnesium sulfate, if given as a bolus, helps to raise the shivering threshold. Rapid-acting anesthetics may also be used, especially neuromuscular blocking agents such as cisatracurium.

Hemodynamics are affected because TH causes hypertension and sinus tachycardia in the initial phase due to cutaneous vasoconstriction. Once TH is achieved, however, sinus bradycardia is the most common arrhythmia.

Hyperglycemia is commonly seen during TH because lower temperatures will decrease insulin secretion and increase insulin resistance. TH can cause hypokalemia by increasing potassium influx into the cells, and rewarming reverses this process.

The most common infections seen in patients with SCA are related to lung infections, especially due to mechanical ventilation.

Trouble Shooting

Once TH is initiated, ice packs and cooling blankets can be used during the rapid initiation with temperature-regulated cooling devices to maintain target temperatures. Temperature fluctuations should be minimized to less than 0.5°C during the maintenance phase.

Mechanical Cardiopulmonary Resuscitation Devices

Introduction

Early CPR has been shown to improve survival in patients with SCA. However, manual compressions are subject to human error, especially rescuer fatigue, which affects CPR quality. Mechanical CPR devices are automated and provide continuous chest compressions during SCA. They are gradually replacing manual compressions, which remain the standard of care (see Tables 1-2 and 1-3).

There are 2 main types of mechanical CPR devices, **pneumatic piston devices and load-distributing band devices.**

■ **TABLE 1-2. AHA Guideline Statement**

Recommendations for Mechanical CPR Devices

COR	LOE	Recommendations
2b	C-LD	1. The use of mechanical CPR devices may be considered in specific settings where the delivery of high-quality manual compressions may be challenging or dangerous for the provider, as long as rescuers strictly limit interruptions in CPR during deployment and removal of the device.
3: No Benefit	B-R	2. The routine use of mechanical CPR devices is not recommended.

Abbreviations: COR, class of recommendation; LOE, level of evidence.

Lucas, the most common device, is a pneumatic piston device that can be used only in adults (Figure 1-6). It works by creating an active decompression suction on the upstroke. It is portable and easy to fit with a small backboard that can be placed under most patients.

AutoPulse device has a load-distributing compression band that will compress the entire thorax. It can only be used in patients who weigh less than 130 kg (Figure 1-7).

Advantages of Mechanical CPR Devices

Advantages include the following:

- Consistent quality of chest compressions
- Safe defibrillation
- Decreased interruption from a change of personnel or exhaustion
- Can facilitate percutaneous coronary intervention and initiation of extracorporeal membrane oxygenation (ECMO) during CPR

Despite the advantages, mechanical CPR has not been found to be superior to manual compression in major trials such as CIRC, LINC, and ParaMeDiC. Besides the availability and economic issues, it requires staff training and can be ineffective for certain body habitus. It is also associated with more patient trauma and is not suitable for the pediatric population.

■ **TABLE 1-3.** Resuscitation Guidance[1]

Invasive Method	Noninvasive Method
Arterial line waveform If arterial line present, coronary perfusion pressure (DBP-RAP) to keep DBP 30-40 and CPP 15 mmHg for organ perfusion. **Central venous oxygen saturation** Continuous oximetry in SVC to target SvO_2 above 30% is desirable for ROSC.	**Echocardiography (TTE OR TEE)** Visual assessment of cardiac motion during CPR is an effective way of achieving ROSC. **End-tidal CO_2 measurement** • It is the amount of CO_2 exhaled in each breath, with normal range 35-40 mmHg. • It can be assessed by waveform or colorimetric method. • Colorimetric method is used for ETT placement with some limitations. • Waveform capnography can detect real-time effective CPR and ROSC. If it is <20 mmHg, CPR needs to be effective, and once it is >40 mmHg, ROSC is achieved.

[1]Effective resuscitation can be guided by invasive or noninvasive methods.

Abbreviations: CPP, coronary perfusion pressure; DBP, diastolic blood pressure; RAP, right atrial pressure; SVC, superior vena cava; TEE, transesophageal echocardiography; TTE, transthoracic echocardiography.

Indications

Mechanical CPR devices are indicated in adult patients for external cardiac compressions who have an acute cardiac arrest in absence of spontaneous breathing and pulse and loss of consciousness. (See Figure 1-8.)

It is used as an adjunct to manual CPR when effective manual CPR is not possible, such as when transporting patients, with insufficient personnel, and with fatigue.

Contraindications

A contraindication is if it is not possible to position the Lucas safely and correctly on the chest of the patient. It is also not possible to place the device in a very small or very large patient.

Trouble Shooting

Before usage, it is important to make sure that the Lucas device is checked and ready for use because batteries need to be charged for at least 4 hours. The battery indicator shows the battery charge status. Some

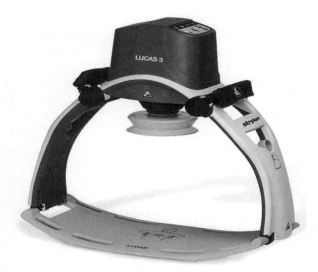

FIGURE 1-6. Lucas device.

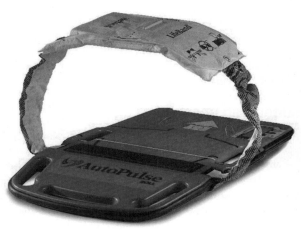

FIGURE 1-7. AutoPulse device.

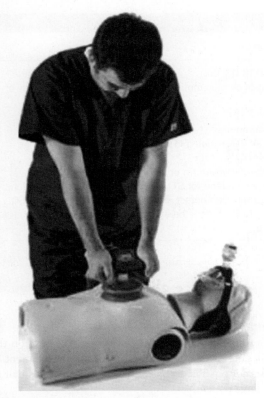

FIGURE 1-8. Mechanical CPR positioning.

other issues include the appropriate attachment of the suction cup to the piston and the correct placement of the patient straps.

■ FUTURE DIRECTIONS

- Efforts have been ongoing to incorporate artificial intelligence in resuscitation care with use of updated algorithms and mobile applications.
- Refresher courses and public awareness for bystander CPR are being encouraged at the grassroots level.

SUGGESTED READINGS

Armstrong L, Caulkett N, Boysen S, Pearson JM, Knight CG, Windeyer MC. Assessing the efficacy of ventilation of anesthetized neonatal calves using a laryngeal mask airway or mask resuscitator. *Front Vet Sci.* 2018;5:292.

De Rosa S, Messina A, Sorbello M, et al. Laryngeal mask airway supreme vs. the Spritztube tracheal cannula in anaesthetised adult patients: a randomised controlled trial. *Eur J Anaesthesiol.* 2019;36(12):955-962.

In CB, Cho SA, Lee SJ, Sung TY, Cho CK. Comparison of the clinical performance of airway management with the i-gel® and laryngeal mask airway Supreme™ in geriatric patients: a prospective and randomized study. *Korean J Anesthesiol.* 2019;72(1):39-46.

Kim HY, Baek SH, Cho YH, et al. Iatrogenic intramural dissection of the esophagus after insertion of a laryngeal mask airway. *Acute Crit Care.* 2018;33(4):276-279.

Klučka J, Šenkyřík J, Skotáková J, et al. Laryngeal mask airway Unique™ position in paediatric patients undergoing magnetic resonance imaging (MRI): prospective observational study. *BMC Anesthesiol.* 2018;18(1):153.

Otten D, Liao MM, Wolken R, et al. Comparison of bag-valve-mask hand-sealing techniques in a simulated model. *Ann Emerg Med.* 2014;63(1):6-12.e3.

Sabuncu U, Kusderci HS, Oterkus M, et al. AuraGain and i-Gel laryngeal masks in general anesthesia for laparoscopic cholecystectomy. Performance characteristics and effects on hemodynamics. *Saudi Med J.* 2018;39(11):1082-1089.

Singh A, Bhalotra AR, Anand R. A comparative evaluation of ProSeal laryngeal mask airway, I-gel and Supreme laryngeal mask airway in adult patients undergoing elective surgery: a randomised trial. *Indian J Anaesth.* 2018;62(11):858-864.

Soleimanpour M, Rahmani F, Ala A, et al. Comparison of four techniques on facility of two-hand bag-valve-mask (BVM) ventilation: E-C, thenar eminence, thenar eminence (dominant hand)-E-C (non-dominant hand) and thenar eminence (non-dominant hand) - E-C (dominant hand). *J Cardiovasc Thorac Res.* 2016;8(4):147-151.

Strametz R, Bergold MN, Weberschock T. Laryngeal mask airway versus endotracheal tube for percutaneous dilatational tracheostomy in critically ill adults. *Cochrane Database Syst Rev.* 2018;11(11):CD009901.

White L, Melhuish T, Holyoak R, Ryan T, Kempton H, Vlok R. Advanced airway management in out of hospital cardiac arrest: a systematic review and meta-analysis. *Am J Emerg Med.* 2018;36(12):2298-2306.

Abbreviations

ACLS: Advanced cardiac life support
AED: Automated external defibrillation
AHA: American Heart Association
BVM: Bag valve mask
CICU: Cardiac intensive care unit
CPR: Cardiopulmonary resuscitation
DES: Drug-eluting stent
DNR: Do not resuscitate
DMT2: Diabetes mellitus type 2
ECG: Electrocardiogram

ECMO: Extracorporeal mechanical oxygenation
EMS: Emergency medical service
$EtCO_2$: End-tidal carbon dioxide
ETT: Endotracheal tube
FM: Face-mask
GA: Gross airway
HEENT: Head, eyes, ears, nose, and throat
HTN: Hypertension
ICH: Intracranial hemorrhage
ICU: Intensive care unit

LAD: Left anterior descending
LMA: Laryngeal mask airway
OR: Operating room
PEEP: Positive end-expiratory pressure
PPV: Positive-pressure ventilation
ROSC: Return of spontaneous circulation
SCA: Sudden cardiac arrest
TH: Therapeutic hypothermia
VF: Ventricular fibrillation
VT: Ventricular tachycardia

CHAPTER 2

Valvular and Structural Heart Devices

• *Jeirym Miranda, MD; Wajiha Jahangir, MD*

■ CASE PRESENTATION

History of Present Illness: A 75-year-old Hispanic elderly man with multiple comorbidities presented to the emergency department (ED) with complaints of shortness of breath and decreased exercise tolerance that had been progressively worsened over the past 4 months. Prior to this presentation, he had recurrent admission due to similar complaints. He was being evaluated at an ambulatory cardiology clinic for an elective valvular intervention after being recently diagnosed with severe aortic stenosis and heart failure with reduced ejection fraction (HFrEF).

Past Medical History: Past medical history includes severe chronic obstructive pulmonary disease (COPD), type 2 diabetes mellitus, pulmonary embolism and recently diagnosed nonischemic cardiomyopathy, heart failure with severely reduced left ventricular (LV) systolic function (HFrEF), New York Heart Association (NYHA)/American College of Cardiology (ACC) class III/stage C and valvular heart disease (VHD)/severe aortic valve stenosis, and moderate mitral valve regurgitation.

Investigations: Initial laboratory findings revealed respiratory acidosis and leukocytosis with a white blood cell (WBC) count of 26,000/mm^3 with a left-sided shift; however, infective workup was negative. He had a hemoglobin of 12.8 g/dL and platelets of 342 mmol/liter. At presentation, laboratory results were as follows: lactate 3.9 mmol/liter, potassium 5.3 mEq/dL, sodium 140 mEq/dL, glucose 187 mg/dL, creatinine 1.3 mg/dL, glomerular filtration rate (GFR) 42.5 mL/min, blood urea nitrogen (BUN) 34 mg/dL, and pro–B-type natriuretic peptide (BNP) 12,333 pg/min. A 12-lead electrocardiogram showed a normal sinus rhythm with marked LV hypertrophy and nonspecific ST-segment changes. A chest X-ray revealed emphysematous changes with significant vascular congestion and increasing consolidation of the lung fields. Earlier investigations including a transthoracic echocardiogram (TTE) showed severely decreased LV ejection fraction (EF) of 25% with restrictive pattern of diastolic dysfunction and increased filling pressure. There was mild aortic regurgitation and severe calcific aortic valve stenosis with an average peak velocity of 4.4 cm/s, mean gradient of 42 mmHg, dimensionless valve index (DVI) of 0.22, and aortic valve area (AVA) by continuity 0.44 cm^2. On mitral valve, moderate mitral annular calcification (MAC) was noted with moderate mitral valve regurgitation. Right-sided structures and function were normal except for moderately elevated pulmonary artery pressure. These findings were similar in a subsequently performed transesophageal echocardiogram (TEE). The patient had previously undergone coronary evaluation with a left heart catheterization, which showed nonobstructive disease with moderate disease involving the left anterior descending and circumflex arteries.

Management: Given hypoxemia and hemodynamic instability, the patient was admitted to the cardiac intensive care unit and was treated for acute-on-chronic hypercapnic and hypoxic respiratory failure secondary to pulmonary edema with superimposed pneumonia and COPD. Broad-spectrum antibiotics were initiated, as well as diuretics and phenylephrine for hemodynamic support in view of developing cardiogenic shock. Later, he required intubation with mechanical ventilation and experienced acute kidney injury and atrial fibrillation with rapid ventricular response. After heart team discussion, given multiple baseline comorbidities, recurrent admissions for heart failure (HF), and worsening clinical status despite medical therapy, he was deemed intermediate to high risk for surgical intervention of the aortic valve (Society of Thoracic Surgeons [STS] score: 7.5%), and the patient was transferred to a quaternary center for urgent transcatheter aortic valve replacement (TAVR).

While undergoing preprocedural evaluation, the patient was successfully extubated. Preprocedure planning imaging including cardiac and abdominal pelvic computed tomography (CT) and angiography revealed normal cardiac anatomy with severe aortic calcium score of 3135 and no significant aortopathy or vascular tortuosity that might have precluded transcatheter intervention on planned access via femoral approach. The patient was taken to the operating room and underwent anesthesia. After being prepped and draped in the usual sterile fashion, a radial arterial and central line was placed. Percutaneous access was obtained in both femoral arteries. A temporary transvenous pacing (TVP) wire was placed in the right ventricle. A guidewire and pigtail were placed into the ascending aorta. A confirmatory aortogram was performed showing the 3 sinuses and their outer angles confirmed by CT scan for optimizing visualization of the sinuses and the annulus. After being adequately anticoagulated, a 14-F sheath was placed into the right groin, a 6-F sheath was contralaterally placed into the left groin, and the guidewire was paced through the aortic valve into the LV. A 29-mm Medtronic Evolut CoreValve was loaded and advanced into position. The patient was rapidly paced at 120 bpm and tolerated the pacing with return of blood pressure. The valve was finely adjusted at the annulus and then deployed with pacing at 120 and under direct fluoroscopy. Selective aortogram and TTE showed trivial paravalvular leak. The delivery system was removed. Final angiogram confirmed that the iliac arteries were patent with no evidence of dissection or leak.

All the sheaths and guidewires were removed, and hemostasis of both femoral arteries was achieved with Perclose device. Hemostasis of the groin was obtained. The patient did not require pacing; therefore, TVP was removed. The patient was transferred to recovery in stable condition. A postprocedure TTE demonstrated a normal-functioning TAVR valve without paravalvular leak. Vascular Doppler showed no evidence of pseudoaneurysms, hematomas, or arteriovenous (AV) fistulas. Postoperative hospital course was uncomplicated, and the patient was successfully discharged home. After several months of follow-up, the patient reported doing clinically well and reportedly was back to baseline functional status without further hospitalizations.

■ KEY POINTS

- Multimodality imaging is recommended to guide the management of any valvular dysfunction including native or prosthetic heart valves, with a TTE as first line, followed by TEE, cardiac CT, magnetic resonance imaging (MRI), and right and left heart catheterization, if clinically indicated.

- Bioprosthetic or repaired native valve dysfunction will typically present with sudden onset of HF symptoms or a change in the auscultatory findings, and these symptoms may be more severe and abrupt in case of infective endocarditis or rupture of valve cups.

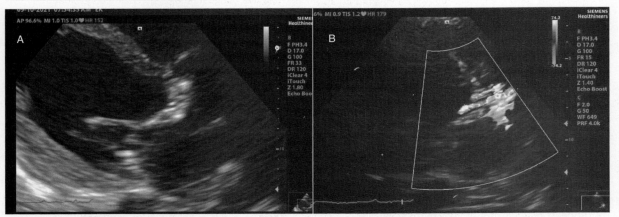

FIGURE 2-1. A. Parasternal long axis (PLAX) view with severe calcific aortic valve, moderate mitral annular calcification, and dilated left ventricular cavity. **B.** Color Doppler on aortic valve showing flow acceleration suggestive of aortic stenosis. (See color insert.)

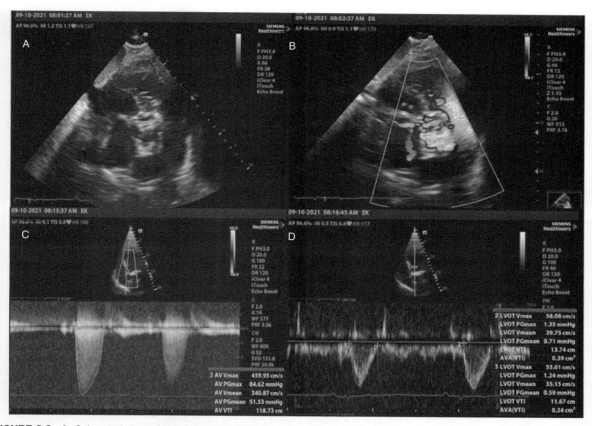

FIGURE 2-2. A. Subcostal view of the aortic valve, which is echo dense with decreased leaflet opening and severe aortic stenosis (AS). **B.** Subcostal view of the aortic valve with flow acceleration on color Doppler. **C.** Continuous Doppler across aortic valve with an average peak velocity of 4 m/s. **D.** Calculated aortic valve area (AVA) by continuity of 0.4 cm². (See color insert.)

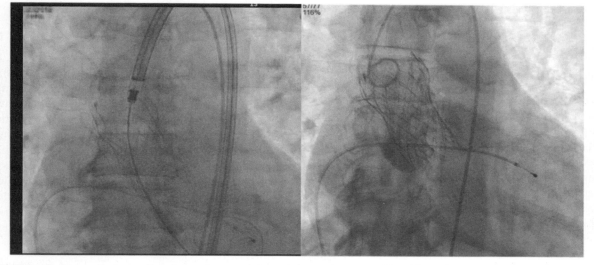

FIGURE 2-3. Transcatheter aortic valve replacement through femoral access with a 29-mm Medtronic Evolut CoreValve.

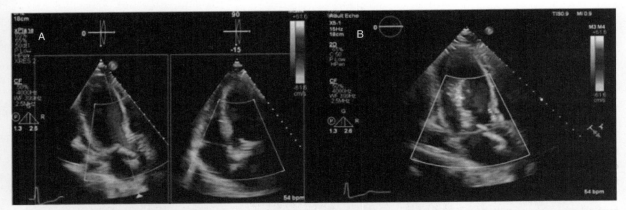

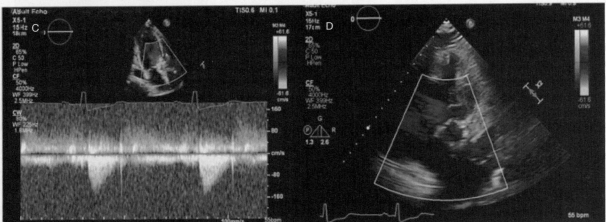

FIGURE 2-4. Post–transcatheter aortic valve replacement (TAVR) 3-chamber echocardiographic view with color Doppler on left ventricular outflow tract (LVOT) and prosthetic valve without evidence of stenosis **(A)** and trace paravalvular leak **(B)**. **C.** Decreased velocities through aortic valve post-TAVR. **D.** Subcostal view with color Doppler on aortic valve post-TAVR showing no stenosis or paravalvular leak (PVL). (See color insert.)

■ INTRODUCTION

Valvular heart disease (VHD) is one of the most common causes of admission to the cardiac intensive unit, especially when developing acutely or after decompensation of a known valvulopathy that is frequently complicated by cardiogenic shock (CS). VHD, including valvular regurgitation and stenosis, is commonly secondary to acute coronary syndrome (ACS); heart failure (HF); aging; degenerative, congenital, or rheumatic heart disease; endocarditis; trauma; or iatrogenic disease. Depending on the severity of symptoms and the patient's clinical status, an emergent or urgent surgical intervention is required to improve outcome when medical therapy alone is not feasible. The vast majority of patients in cardiac care units usually have multiple related comorbidities including HF, arrhythmias, ischemic cardiomyopathy, and concomitant other valvular disease, which in addition to their acute illness, will place these patients at a significant increased risk for surgical intervention. Due to new advances, we have numerous transcatheter and percutaneous valvular devices used for temporary stabilization or as long-term management of these high-risk patients when a surgical approach is contraindicated or prohibited.

For acute settings, unfortunately, there are not enough data or clinical guidelines to support the indication or timing of a percutaneous or transcatheter approach, and most of the available devices are still undergoing investigation with only a few being US Food and Drug Administration (FDA) approved. One must keep in mind that in acute settings the severity and hemodynamic assessment of any valvular disease might be challenging and can be affected by extreme loading conditions and use of inotropes and vasopressors. It is also important to determine if the valvular disease is the only responsible factor causing the patient's current status or if it might be driven by another pathology that can sometimes be reversible.

Multimodality imaging is recommended to guide the management of any valvular dysfunction including native or prosthetic heart valves, with transthoracic echocardiogram (TTE) as the first line, followed by transesophageal echocardiogram (TEE), cardiac computed tomography (CT), magnetic resonance imaging (MRI), and right and left heart catheterization, if clinically indicated. Therefore, when evaluating any patient in a cardiac unit for a less invasive approach, an extensive heart team discussion is mandatory with a detailed assessment of the patient's candidacy, including valvular anatomy, the etiology and mechanism of the disease, and determining the most appropriate approach considering underlying comorbidities, possible peri-intervention complications, postoperative care, and the patient's long-term goals and outcome.

In this chapter, some available devices are discussed, including indications, contraindications, mechanism, and potential complications.

■ MITRAL VALVE DISEASE AND TRANSCATHETER INTERVENTION

The prevalence of moderate or severe mitral valve disease in patients 75 years old or older in the United States is approaching approximately 10%. Mitral diseases can be divided into mitral stenosis (MS) and mitral regurgitation (MR), according to different hemodynamics. MS is more prevalent in developing countries, mostly resulting from rheumatic infection, with similar results in surgical or percutaneous balloon mitral valvuloplasty (BMV) treatment in this population. MR is a worldwide frequent valvulopathy and it can be divided into organic or primary and functional or secondary lesions.[1]

■ MITRAL REGURGITATION

The pathophysiology of MR is characterized by changes in ventricular loading that cause dilation of the left ventricle (LV), dysfunction, and subsequently HF.[2] TTE should be the initial imaging modality for the evaluation and screening of all mitral valve morphology and pathology, which can aid in the determination of mechanism and quantification of MR severity, as well as assessment of left-sided chamber size and function. Some parameters used to assess MR include a 2-dimensional assessment of mitral valve leaflet motion, thickness, coaptation, the MR jet to left atrial (LA) area ratio, effective regurgitant orifice area (EROA), vena contracta, regurgitant area, regurgitant volume, LV ejection fraction (LVEF), and LV end-diastolic area (LVEDA). When the images from TTE are inadequate, a TEE can provide the information and assessment. Three-dimensional TEE can provide an "enface" view of the mitral valve that resembles surgical inspection, facilitating preprocedure planning. Other modalities like cardiac MRI can provide accurate information of MR and LV dimensions when TEE is contraindicated.[3]

Severe MR in the CS setting becomes a complex situation requiring in most cases the combination of optimal medical management with inotropic agents, airway intubation, and mechanical support to improve hemodynamic tolerance of MR. Distinguishing primary from function MR is essential before considering an interventional approach.[4] Surgical treatment can lead to improvements of symptoms, LV remodeling, and survival in selected patients, whether MR is primary or secondary.[2] Although surgery is considered the gold-standard treatment for primary MR, for secondary MR, because it is associated with evolved ventricular disease, there are no sufficient data supporting the value of surgery and valvular interventionin this type of MR and it may be considered only when symptoms are severe and persistent despite medical therapy.[4]

Many of these patients have a very high perioperative risk, and percutaneous management may be feasible; however, it remains experimental. In comparison to the aortic valve, the mitral valve pathology is more complex, involving the valve leaflets and sometimes the annulus, which makes the transcatheter repair process much more challenging. Percutaneous interventions can be divided into transcatheter edge-to-edge leaflet repair, annuloplasty, mitral valve replacement, and other miscellaneous approaches.[3,7] (See Table 2-1 and Figure 2-5.)

■ TABLE 2-1. Transcatheter Mitral Valve Devices

Device	Manufacture	Access size sheath	Anchoring mechanism	Valve size
Tendyne	Abbott	TA 34 Fr.	Apical tether	Outer (sealing) frame ranges 30–43 mm in the SL dimension and 34–50 in the IC dimension
Intrepid	Medtronic	TA 33Fr.	Radial force and sub-annular cleats	Inner stent–27 mm (Outer stent–43, 46, and 50 mm)
TIARA	Neovasc	TA 32, 36 Fr.	3 ventricular anchoring tabs (onto the fibrous trigone and posterior shelf of the annulus)	35 and 40 mm
CardiaQ	Edwards Lifesciences	TA/TF 33 Fr.	Mitral annulus capture with native leaflet engagement	30 mm
Sapiens M3	Edwards Lifesciences	TF/TA 20 Fr.	Nitinol dock system	29
Caisson	LivaNova	TF 31 Fr.	4 sub-annular anchoring feet 3 atrial holding features	36A 42A 42B
HighLife	HighLife SAS	TA39 Fr. (TF artery for loop placement)	External anchor; valve in sub-annular mitral ring	31 mm
Fortis	Edwards Lifesciences	TA 42 Fr.	2 opposing paddles	29 mm
CardioValve	CardioValve	TF 28-Fr.	24 focal "sandwiching" points	3 sizes (range 40–40 mm)
Evoque	Edwards Lifesciences	TF 28-Fr.	External anchor	2 sizes (44 and 48 mm)

Fr, French; TA, transapical; TF, transfemoral.

Source: Reproduced from Gheorghe L, et al. Current Devices in Mitral Valve Replacement and Their Potential Complications. *Front Cardiovasc Med.* 2020;7:531843, Table 2.[10]

Effective orifice area	Valve position	Recapture	Shape	Frame	Leaflets
3.2 cm^2	Intra-annular	Fully recapturable system after complete deployment	D-shaped (outer stent) Circular (inner frame)	Nitinol, double frame; Self-expandable	Porcine pericardium, trileaflet
2.4 cm^2	Intra-annular	No	Circular	Double stent, self-expanding, nitinol	Bovine pericardium, trileaflet
6.5–12 cm^2	Intra-annular	No	D-shaped	Self-expanding, nitinol	Bovine pericardium, trileaflet
NA	Supra-annular	No	Circular	Self-expanding, nitinol	Bovine pericardium, trileaflet
NA	Intra-annular	No	Circular	Balloon-expandable, cobalt-chromium frame	Bovine pericardium, trileaflet
NA	Supra-annular	Recapturable/ retrievable	D-shaped	2 components (anchor and valve); Nitinol, self-expandable.	Porcine Pericardium, trileaflet
NA	Intra-annular	No	Circular	2 components (ring and valve); Nitinol, self-expandable	Bovine pericardium, trileaflet
NA	Intra-annular	No	Circular	Cloth-covered, self-expanding, nitinol	Bovine pericardium, trileaflet
NA	Intra-annular	No	Circular	Dual nitinol frame	Bovine pericardium, trileaflet
NA	Intra-annular	No	Circular	Self-expanding, nitinol with fabric skirt to minimize paravalvular leak	Bovine pericardium, trileaflet

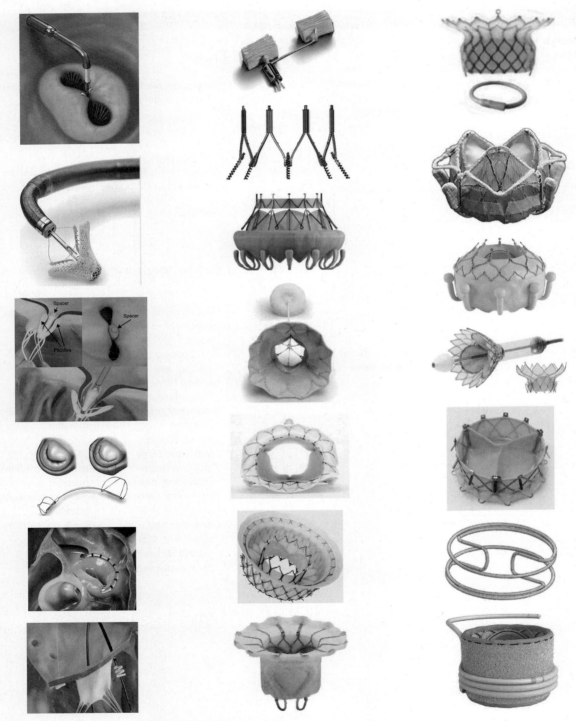

FIGURE 2-5. Illustration of mitral valve transcatheter devices. (See color insert.)

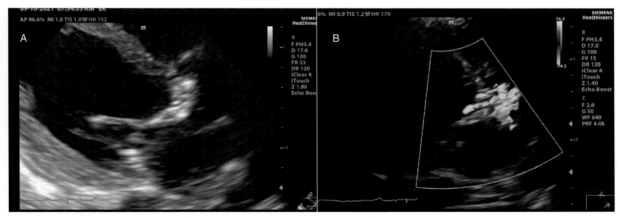

FIGURE 2-1. A. Parasternal long axis (PLAX) view with severe calcific aortic valve, moderate mitral annular calcification, and dilated left ventricular cavity. **B.** Color Doppler on aortic valve showing flow acceleration suggestive of aortic stenosis.

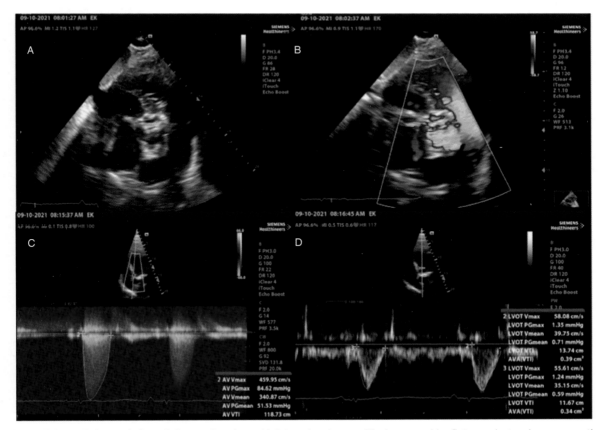

FIGURE 2-2. A. Subcostal view of the aortic valve, which is echo dense with decreased leaflet opening and severe aortic stenosis (AS). **B.** Subcostal view of the aortic valve with flow acceleration on color Doppler. **C.** Continuous Doppler across aortic valve with an average peak velocity of 4 m/s. **D.** Calculated aortic valve area (AVA) by continuity of 0.4 cm^2.

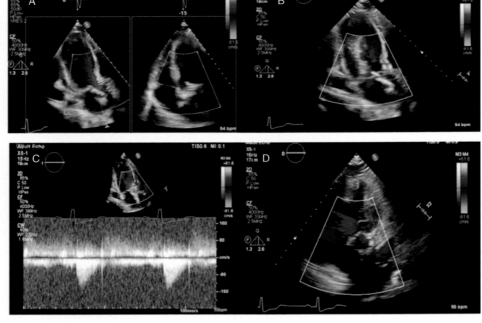

FIGURE 2-4. Post–transcatheter aortic valve replacement (TAVR) 3-chamber echocardiographic view with color Doppler on left ventricular outflow tract (LVOT) and prosthetic valve without evidence of stenosis **(A)** and trace paravalvular leak **(B).** **C.** Decreased velocities through aortic valve post-TAVR. **D.** Subcostal view with color Doppler on aortic valve post-TAVR showing no stenosis or paravalvular leak (PVL).

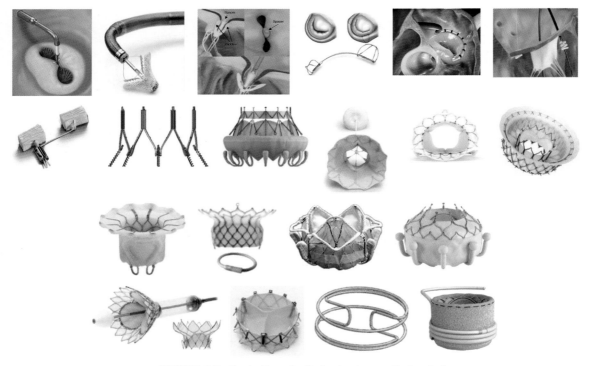

FIGURE 2-5. Illustration of mitral valve transcatheter devices.

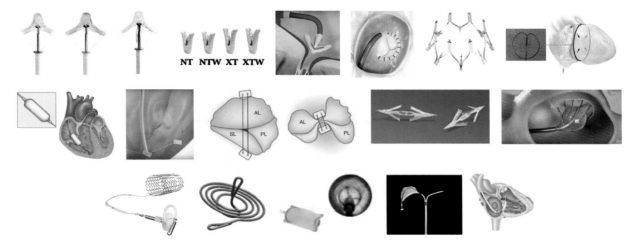

FIGURE 2-6. Current devices for transcatheter tricuspid valve repair.

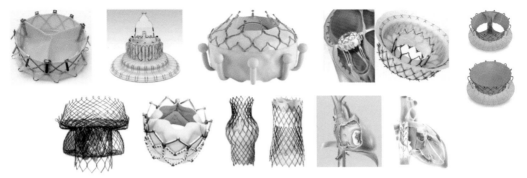

FIGURE 2-7. Transcatheter tricuspid valve replacement.

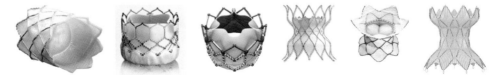

FIGURE 2-8. Transcatheter pulmonary valves.

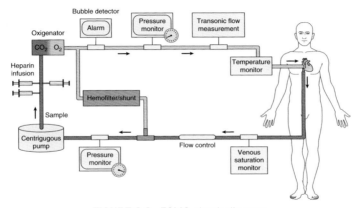

FIGURE 3-6. ECMO circuit diagram.

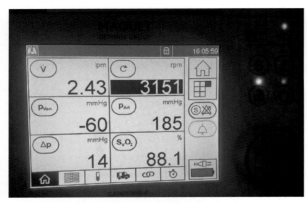

FIGURE 3-7. ECMO console in coronary care unit patient.

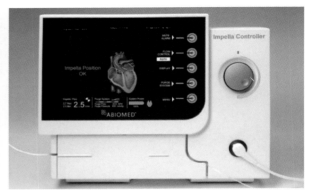

FIGURE 4-5. Impella controller.

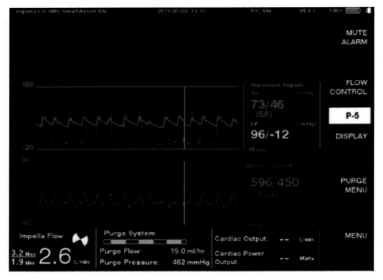

FIGURE 4-6. Placement screen.

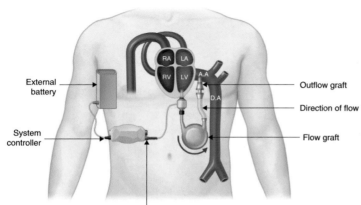

FIGURE 5-5. LVAD configuration.

External battery

System controller

Percutaneous lead

Outflow graft

Direction of flow

Flow graft

FIGURE 5-6. SynCardia. (From SynCardia Systems, Tucson, Arizona.)

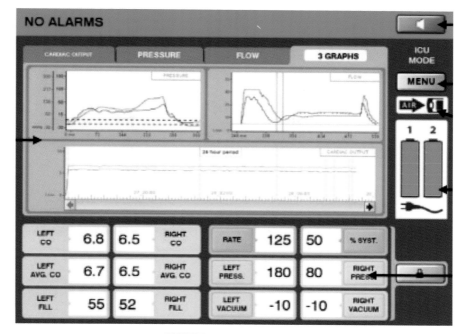

FIGURE 5-7. TAH interface.

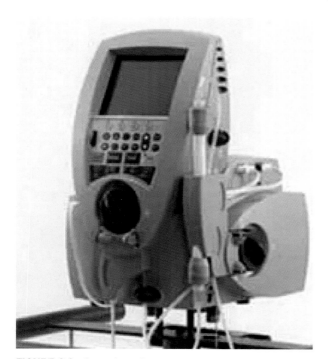

FIGURE 6-9. Aquapheresis setup.

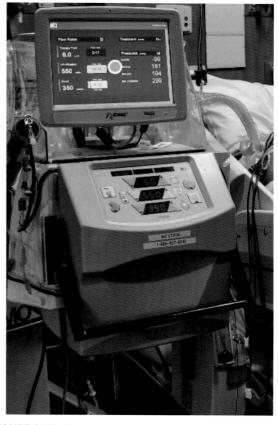

FIGURE 6-10. Continuous venovenous hemofiltration setup.

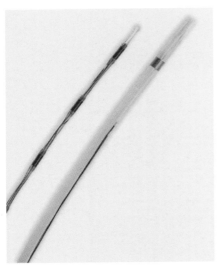

FIGURE 7-2. EKOS catheter used for CDT.

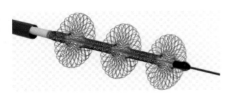

FIGURE 7-4. Inari FlowTriever catheter.

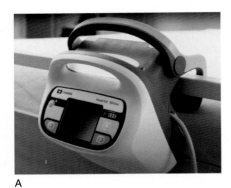

A

B

FIGURE 7-7. A, B. Pneumatic compression device.

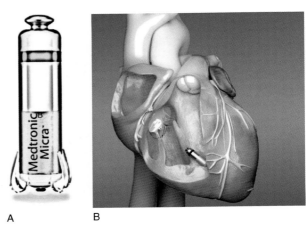

A

B

FIGURE 8-4. A, B. Leadless pacemaker. The blue arrow shows the implanted leadless pacemaker.

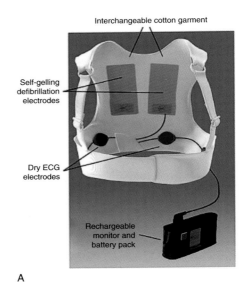

Interchangeable cotton garment

Self-gelling defibrillation electrodes

Dry ECG electrodes

Rechargeable monitor and battery pack

A

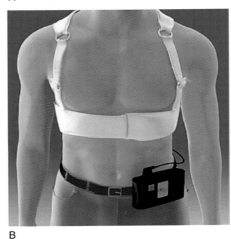

B

FIGURE 8-8. A, B. Wearable cardioverter defibrillator (Life Vest).

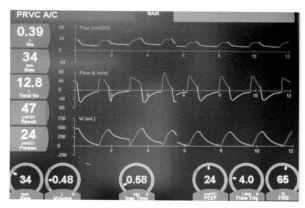

FIGURE 9-5. Parameter display on MV.

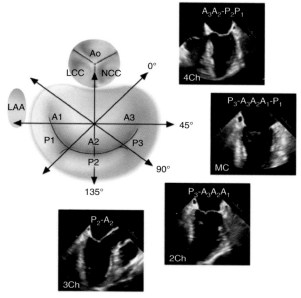

FIGURE 10-13. Views of TEE. Ao aorta; LAA, left atrial appendage; LCC, left coronary cusp; NCC, noncoronary cusp. (Reproduced with permission from Hahn RT, Abraham T, Adams MS, Bruce CJ, Glas KE, Lang RM, Reeves ST, Shanewise JS, Siu SC, Stewart W, Picard MH. Guidelines for performing a comprehensive transesophageal echocardiographic examination: recommendations from the American Society of Echocardiography and the Society of Cardiovascular Anesthesiologists. *J Am Soc Echocardiogr.* 2013;26(9):921-64.)

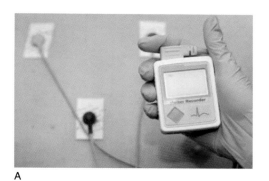

A

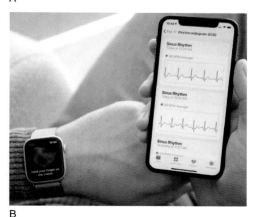

B

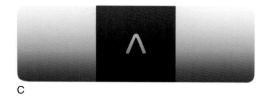

C

FIGURE 10-3. A-C. Various types of heart rate monitors.

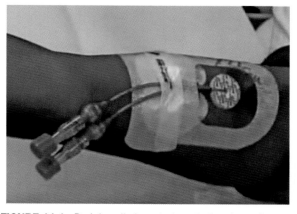

FIGURE 11-1. Peripherally inserted central catheter line.

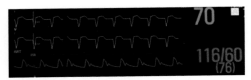

FIGURE 11-2. Arterial line waveform.

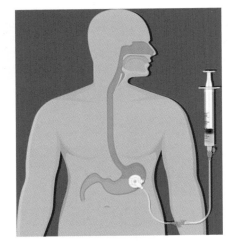

FIGURE 11-6. Gastrostomy tube (G-tube).

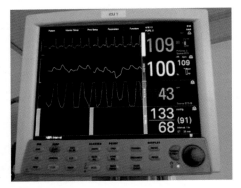

FIGURE 12-1. Bedside blood pressure monitor (oscilloscope).

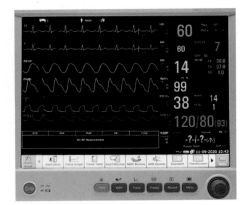

FIGURE 12-2. Bedside monitor.

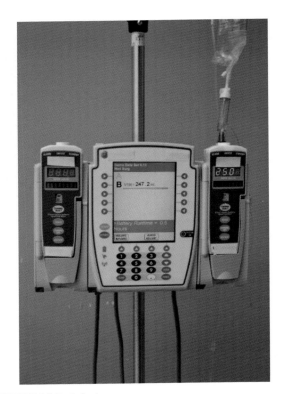

FIGURE 12-5. Infusion pump.

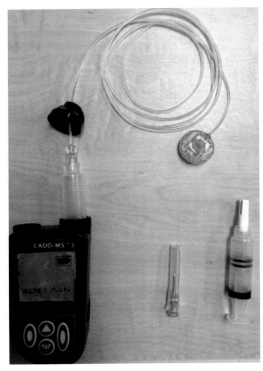

FIGURE 12-6. Remodulin subcutaneous pump.

Summary of Current Percutaneous Mitral Valve Repair Devices and Technique Currently in Evolution

- Edge-to-Edge Repair
  a. MitraClip* (Abbott Vascular, Abbott Park, IL)
  b. PASCAL (Edwards Lifesciences, Irvine, CA)
  c. Valve clamp
  d. Mitral stitch
- Annuloplasty
  a. Cardioband (Edwards Lifesciences, Irvine, CA)
  b. Millipede IRIS (Millipede, Santa Rosa, CA)
  c. Carillon (Cardiac Dimensions, Kirkland, WA)
  d. ARTO (MVRx, San Mateo, CA)
  e. AccuCinch (Ancora Heart, Santa Clara, CA)
  f. Amend (Valcare Medical, Herzlyia Pituach, Israel)
  g. Mitral cerclage
- Mitral Valve Replacement
  a. Tendyne (Abbott Vascular, Santa Clara, CA)
  b. Tiara (Neovasc, Richmond, British Columbia, Canada)
  c. EVOQUE (Edwards Lifesciences, Irvine, CA)
  d. Intrepid (Medtronic, Minneapolis, MN)
  e. Caisson (Caisson Interventional LLC; Maple Grove, MN)
  f. HighLife (HighLife Medical, Irvine, CA)
  g. CardiAQ (Edwards Lifesciences, Irvine, CA)
  h. MValve (Boston Scientific, Marlborough, MA)
  i. SAPIEN M3 (Edwards Lifesciences, Irvine, CA)
  j. NAVI (NaviGate Cardiac Structures, Lake Forest, CA)
  k. AltaValve (4C Medical Technologies, Maple Grove, MN)
- Other Approaches
  a. NeoChord DS1000 (NeoChord, St. Louis Park, MN)
  b. Harpoon TDS-5 (Edwards Lifesciences, Irvine, CA)
  c. ChordArt (CoreMedic, Tübingen, Germany)
  d. V-Chordal (Valtech Cardio, Or-Yehuda, Israel)
  e. Pipeline (Gore Medical; Newark, DE)
  f. CardioMech (CardioMech, Trondheim, Norway)
  g. Mitral Butterfly (Angel Valve Vienna, Vienna, Austria)

Mitral Valve "Edge-to-Edge" Transcatheter Repair

MitraClip

To date, the MitraClip (Abbott Vascular, Menlo Park, California) is the most adopted technology and is currently the only FDA approved edge-to-edge technology, being used in nearly 20,000 high-risk or inoperable patients

around the world. In the Endovascular Valve Edge-to-Edge Repair (EVEREST) Study, when compared with surgical repair, the MitraClip had a superior safety profile, mostly based on a lower risk of transfusions. In recent registries, the procedural success has significantly increased, with a reduction in residual MR and improvement of New York Heart Association (NYHA) functional class and quality of life. It has been also studied for secondary MR, with favorable results in terms of mortality and HF hospitalizations compared with optimal medical therapy in the COAPT trial. In the MITRA-FR trial, the results were not as favorable. Due to the absence of data supporting the use of the MitraClip technology in the acute setting, patients who were hemodynamically unstable or in CS were excluded from these studies. Thus, the management of acute MR in CS with a MitraClip placement remains experimental but has been considered in some reported cases as an acceptable rescue option, after a precise assessment of anatomic valve characteristics and the feasibility of the approach.[4,5]

Indications

- Moderate to severe organic or primary MR (3 to 4+)
- Severe symptomatic NYHA class III or IV HF
- Nonsurgical candidate (prohibitive risk is defined as a Society of Thoracic Surgeons score predicted risk of mortality of >8% for mitral valve replacement or >6% for mitral valve repair)
- Anatomy favorable for repair (Table 2-2)
- Good life expectancy

Contraindications

- Active endocarditis of the mitral valve
- Rheumatic mitral valve disease
- Severe mitral annular calcification involving leaflets
- Presence of significant cleft or perforation in mitral valve leaflets
- Intracardiac, inferior vena cava (IVC), or femoral venous thrombus
- Unable to tolerate anticoagulation or the necessary postprocedural antiplatelet regimen
- Mitral valve stenosis[3]

Mechanism of Mitral Clip

The device consists of a clip made of cobalt-chromium that reproduces the Alfieri repair, a surgical technique in which sutures opposing leaflets are placed at the site of MR. A multisteering catheter delivered transseptally is

---

*Only MitraClip is Food and Drug Administration approved for use in the United States.

■ **TABLE 2-2. Morphological Characterization for MitraClip Eligibility**

Transcatheter MVR	Feasible		Unlikely
Calcification	None	Annular-sparing grasping zone	Grasping zone
MVA and MV gradient	>4 cm^2 and <4 mm Hg	3.5 – 4 cm^2	<3.5 cm^2 and <5 mm Hg
Flail width	<15 mm	>15 mm	
Flial gap	<10 mm	>10 mm	

directed toward the mitral valve; the clip is then opened and oriented perpendicular to the coaptation line in order to grasp the free edges of the opposing leaflets, creating a double-orifice mitral valve. The device is repositionable and retrievable, and multiple clips can be deployed to achieve optimal results if needed.[5]

Complications

Major adverse event rate with MitraClip has decreased from 15% in 2005 to less than 3.5% in 2020 after technical developments and growing proceduralist experience. Older patients, females, and those with poorer baseline health status typically experience more complications. MitraClip-associated complications can be considered as procedure or device related, including but not limited to the following compliations.[3,6,7] (See Table 2-3.)

Procedure-Related Complications The complications mainly result from a large-lumen access and the transseptal puncture.

Death and need for resuscitation. Although most people treated with MitraClip are usually high-risk patients, real-world data show a very low intraprocedural and in-hospital mortality. The latest studies with the XTR/NTR and G4 reported an even lower in-hospital mortality (XTR/NTR 0.9%, G4 0%).

Access site complications. These can be categorized into vascular and cardiac complications. Vascular complications are more likely associated with the proximity of the femoral vein to the artery and the use of a large-caliber catheter. Studies report rates of 1.4% to 4% for major and 2.7% to 3.8% for minor vascular complications without changes over time. Preprocedural controlled hydration and ultrasound-guided venous puncture are small measures that might decrease vascular complications. Cardiac complications, including pericardial effusion or tamponade (0%-0.5%) and the persistence of iatrogenic atrial septal defect (57%, 50%, and 25% after 1, 6, and 12 months postprocedure,

■ **TABLE 2-3. Complications Related to MitraClip Procedure**

Complication	Management
Pericardial effusion/tamponade	• Can occur due to septal puncture by guidewire or catheter. • Requires emergent drainage
Air embolism	• Can occur due to large sheath • Careful flushing and aspiration is required
Thrombus formation	• Can occur due to wires sheath and prosthetic valves • Need monitoring of act with goal 250-300 sec
Clip detachment from leaflets	• Can occur due to malposition • Need retrieval
Persistent atrial septal defect	• Can occur due to large size mitraclip • Majority of times closes spontaneously but may need intervention if significant shunt present
Chorda tendinea trapped by mitraclip	• Inappropriate positioning • Imaging guided positioning is required
Atrial & ventricular arrythmias	• Related to trigger from catheter • ECG monitoring is required

respectively), are the main access-related cardiac complications and may be reduced by aiming to achieve a posterior and superior position with ultrasound-guided transseptal puncture.

Bleeding complications. These are the most frequent periprocedural complications, with an incidence ranging from 1% to 7.4% depending on the definition and cohort used. Interestingly, a high number of bleeding complications are of gastrointestinal origin and less than 50% are access-related despite the use of large-caliber femoral access. Furthermore, a bleeding history, chronic kidney disease, and coronary artery disease are independent risk factors for bleeding. In addition, most patients receive peri-intervention anticoagulation and/or antiplatelet therapy, if not already included in daily medical regimen, which increases risk of bleeding on access sites.

Thromboembolic events. Overall, major adverse cardiac and cerebrovascular events occurred in real-world data in 3% to 7% of patients, the in-hospital myocardial infarction rate ranges from 0% to 3%, and the incidence of a postprocedural stroke is 0% to 1%. These complications are usually secondary to the use of a large-caliber catheter in the venous system, and the possibility of thrombo- or air-embolic complications must be a serious consideration and may be prevented with adequate anticoagulation, responsible and precise device and catheter handling, and constant flushing.

Acute renal failure. This complication is rare because the implantation procedure itself does not require the administration of contrast medium. Rather, it may be secondary to a systemic inflammatory response due to vascular access or artificial material in the bloodstream or as a consequence from transient hypotension during general anesthesia.

Endocarditis. Mitral valve endocarditis after transcatheter edge-to-edge repair (TEER) is a rare event (0%-2.6%), with only a few cases reported.

Other procedure-related complications. Esophageal injury from intraprocedural TEE, de novo atrial fibrillation, and dislocation of existing pacemaker or defibrillator lead may occur.

Device-Related Complications

Functional device failure. MR reduction will depend on the proceduralist experience to appropriately identify which strategy is optimal for each pathology and to select the most favorable clip size because persistent MR is considered to be an important prognostic factor for rehospitalization and mortality after MitraClip. Wider clip arms and independent grasping are new features of the G4 system and are thought to be responsible for the excellent improvement of procedural results.

Mitral stenosis. Clip-associated MS is associated with higher mortality and worse long-term outcomes. The Mitral Valve Academic Research Consortium (MVARC) defines a postprocedural MS as a mean transvalvular pressure gradient of greater than 5 mmHg. An echocardiographic assessment is crucial before releasing the clip in order to determine the residual MR and MS, and deployment of the clip should be avoided until acceptable gradients are achieved.

Single leaflet device attachment (SLDA). SLDA, which is also known as a single leaflet or partial clip detachment, describes the complete loss of clip connection to one leaflet. It is the most common structural device failure after TEER and may be seen more commonly in complex lesions. This can occur acutely (during the procedure), which is more frequent, or subacutely (first few days after the procedure), whereas late SLDA is infrequent. It is thought that SLDA is caused by insufficient leaflet grasping or by leaflet perforation or tear if SLDA occurs after an adequate grasping.

Clip embolization. Only 2 registries (the Transcatheter Valve Treatment Sentinel Pilot registry [TCVT] and the transcather valve treatment [TVT]) have reported clip embolization with a rate of less than 1%. This rare complication mostly occurs during clip deployment, is immediately recognized, and requires surgical removal.

Leaflet injury/chordae rupture. Isolated leaflet injury has been described in 2% of patients using the third generation of MitraClip device and is mainly caused by repetitive grasping maneuvers performed to achieve a proper device position. Leaflet damage is frequently observed in very thin leaflets or sclerotic valvular annulus with reduced flexibility.[3,6,7]

PASCAL Mitral Valve Repair System

The PASCAL mitral valve repair system uses an edge-to-edge repair technology, similar to MitraClip, despite its rhomboid folding clip structure. The force of clipping and leaflet fixation are based on elastic preformed metal retraction, without additional kinetic work with transseptal approach. The delivery system includes a 22-F guide with both a steerable and an implant catheter. Its implant consists of a central spacer that is designed to fill the regurgitant orifice area and 2 paddles and 2 clasps that allow for independent leaflet capture optimizing its positioning. The multicenter, single-arm, clinical Edwards PASCAL Transcatheter Mitral Valve Repair System study (CLASP) revealed that the overall safety of this device was satisfactory. The device received its CE mark in February 2019, together with the large-scale randomized clinical trial (RCT) CLASP IID/IIF approved by FDA.[1,8]

Transcatheter Mitral Valve Annuloplasty

Indirect Annuloplasty

Indirect annuloplasty reshapes the mitral annulus by using the coronary sinus. Its close proximity allows for device placement that will shorten the posterior annulus, reducing the septal-lateral dimension, followed by a decreased mitral valve orifice area and regurgitation. The Carillon Mitral Contour System (Cardiac Dimensions, Kirkland, Washington) consists of 2 self-expanding nitinol anchors connected by a fixed-length, tension-adjustable cable. Although initial clinical trials (AMADEUS-Mitral Annuloplasty Device European Union Study and TITAN-Transcatheter Implantation of Carillon Mitral Annuloplasty Device and TITAN II trials) have been completed, due to low procedural success rate and risk for coronary sinus dissection and circumflex coronary artery occlusion during deployment, the Carillon only achieved the CE mark and has not progressed to clinical practice use.[1,5]

Direct Annuloplasty

Direct annuloplasty is the most promising approach for transcatheter repair because it can reduce the size of the mitral annulus by placing through a catheter an adjustable prosthetic annulus, reproducing the gold-standard surgical technique. The representative devices are Cardioband (Edwards Lifesciences, Irvine, California) and Mitralign (Mitralign Inc, Tewksbury, Massachusetts). The first-in-man (FIM) study of Mitralign demonstrated a success rate was 70.4% with 50% reduction of MR and significant improvement of cardiac function at 6-month follow-up. The Mitralign system has been designed to perform selective plications in the posterior annulus by deploying couple of transannular pledgeted anchors through an Arterial approach. Tension is applied to sutures connecting the anchors to decrease posterior annular size. The Cardioband system is delivered from a transseptal approach, and a Dacron band is implanted from trigone to trigone using

several annular anchors starting from the anterolateral and progressing to the posteromedial commissure, delivered under echocardiographic and fluoroscopic guidance, with an annular contraction ratio reaching approximately 25% to 30%. Early clinical experience is promising. However, the major limitation of these devices is that they are partial rings. Given this limitation, at present, it is being evaluated in the placement of a complete mitral annuloplasty ring using the Millipede (Millipede, Ann Arbor, Michigan) and enCor (Valcare, Irvine, California) systems.[1,5,8]

Millipede IRIS Complete Annuloplasty Ring This is the first transcatheter, transfemoral, transseptal, semi-rigid, complete annuloplasty ring to be delivered to the mitral valve annulus, mimicking surgical annuloplasty, which is the gold standard for primary MR and functional MR. The device is a semirigid nitinol complete ring that attaches directly to the entire mitral annulus and can normalize the mitral anterior-posterior diameter in patients who are properly selected. The device is supra-annular and does not interfere with the LV outflow tract. Patients had significant reduction in mitral septal-lateral diameter along with significant improvement of MR and NYHA class. In the initial clinical report, it was shown that the Millipede IRIS ring is safe and that there was no device-related procedural death, stroke, or myocardial infarction (MI). Also, it can be used concomitantly with a TEER by the MitraClip device.[8,9]

Transcatheter Mitral Valve Replacement

Although transcatheter mitral valve replacement (TMVR) has been evolving rapidly, when compared to the aortic valve and transcatheter aortic valve replacement (TAVR), TMVR is challenging due to the complexities of the mitral apparatus and concerns including the larger annular size and asymmetrical anatomy, the need for valve anchoring, and the potential for developing LV outflow tract obstruction and paravalvular leak (PVL). In addition, durability issues dealing with stent fracture, tissue erosion, and degeneration require evaluation. An adequate preprocedural study is mandatory and includes multimodality imaging to define the etiology and mechanism of the MR, to determine a patient's eligibility according to anatomic characteristics, to perform implantation access planning, and to identify possible issues during TMVR. TMVR can be divided into valve-in-mitral annular calcification (valve-in-mac), valve-in-native mitral valve (valve-in-valve), and valve-in-degenerated surgical bioprostheses or rings (valve-in-ring), with valve-in-valve having the best performance. Because TMVR remains in the early development stage, there is limited feasibility/ FIM experience. However, newer valve designs such as a D-shaped frame/orifice, self-expanding frame, atrial skirt, and active fixation systems have focused on the procedure challenges.[1,5,10]

After an early FIM TMVR procedure using the Cardi AQ valve (Edwards Lifesciences, Irvine, California) was successfully performed in 2012, new devices have been emerging continuously. These include the Tendyne device (Tendyne Holdings, a subsidiary of Abbott Vascular, Roseville, Minnesota), Neovasc Tiara Device (Neovasc, Richmond, British Columbia, Canada), Intrepid System (Medtronic, Minneapolis, Minnesota), Fortis System (Edwards Lifesciences, Irvine, California), HighLife Device (Peijia Medical Limited Corporation, Suzhou, Jiangsu Province, China), Caisson System (Maple Grove, Minneapolis, Minnesota), MValve Device (Herzliya, Tel Aviv, Israel), and NCS NaviGate System (NaviGate Cardiac Structures, LakeFore St, California).[1,5] (See Table 2-1 and Figure 2-5.)

Complications During and After TMVR

Bleeding. TMVR is associated with high morbidity and mortality, occurring in about 10% to 40% of patients after TMVR due to the transapical approach in most cases. The use of anticoagulation treatment and large-bore access sites (>30 F) may increase bleeding risk despite 2 purse-string sutures with felt pledgets at the access level. The Tendyne valve presents an epicardial pad, which helps to promote hemostasis and reduce the risk of access bleeding. The bleeding rate with the Intrepid procedure was higher, which might be in part due to intensive antiplatelet and anticoagulation therapy after TMVR.

Hemolysis and PVL. Hemolysis is a less frequent complication and may occur after TMVR as a result of turbulent flow pattern and erythrocyte destruction caused by PVL. The incidence of hemolysis and PVLs may be higher in mitral valve-in-ring (MViR) and mitral valve–in–mitral annular calcification (MVi-MAC) because the transcatheter heart valve (THV) does not have the same shape as the native valve/mitral annuloplasty and gaps may remain in between. The treatment can be percutaneous or surgical. However, because these patients are at high risk, surgery remains the last option.

Endocarditis. Reported in the Tendyne, Intrepid, and S3 MViV studies, the rate of endocarditis at 1-year follow-up was 4%. Prophylaxis should be done as for regular bioprosthesis.

Valve thrombogenicity. This may be silent or may present with HF symptoms. It is a serious complication, and the treatment is anticoagulation. The experience with mitral bioprosthesis demonstrated the need for 3 to 6 months of oral anticoagulation after surgical mitral valve replacement to reduce the risk of thromboembolic events (stroke and MI) until the valve is completely endothelialized. Moreover, the turbulent flow around the valve, the preexisting prothrombotic conditions, and new atrial fibrillation can increase the risk of arterial embolism.

Pacemaker implantation. The incidence of pacemaker implantation is approximately 10% to 30%. However, there are no data in the field of TMVR, and it should be hypothetically lower since it does not require predilatation and the valve placement is distant from the septum.

Embolization, migration, malposition. This complication is mainly related to a discordance between the THV and the mitral annulus, previous bioprosthesis, ring, or band. Moreover, there are several THVs with a distinct site of anchoring: at the level of the mitral valve involving the leaflets or not and at the level of the apex or the LA. The absence of calcification and the D-shape in the native valve make a perfect anchoring difficult.[10]

Transcatheter Artificial Chordae Implantation

Transapical off-pump mitral valve repair with NeoChord implantation is a minimally invasive technique that is being applied widely in Europe for mitral valve leaflet prolapse or flail causing severe MR. The NeoChord DS1000 device consists of a high-translucency expanded polytetrafluoroethylene synthetic fiber that is transapically delivered and is used as an artificial chord for mitral valve repair. After gaining access, the delivery system crosses the valve and grasps onto the affected leaflet, confirming the correct position by sending information from the jaws via fiberoptic technology to a designated monitor. The delivery system then pierces the leaflet, delivering the cord and suturing it in place. The chord is thereby secured to the leaflet and then pulled and anchored to the myocardial apex site of entry. The procedure is performed under real-time 2- and 3-dimensional TEE for both implantation and neochordae tension adjustment allowing real-time monitoring of hemodynamic recovery.

This device received its CE mark approval in 2012, and by May 2016, it had received investigational device exemption approval from the FDA.[8,11]

■ MITRAL STENOSIS

The most frequent clinical presentation of MS is HF, which is often associated with atrial fibrillation, and the mortality rate may reach 15% to 20% in pregnant women with severe HF. Medical management is relatively limited in MS patients in CS, and surgery is challenging in this acute setting, especially in pregnancy, as the hemodynamics changes during cardiopulmonary bypass are critical.[4]

BMV was the first catheter-based valvular therapy, described in 1982. When valvular and subvalvular anatomies are favorable, particularly in terms of calcifications, BMV is the cornerstone of treatment for severe MS. In severe calcified degenerative MS, limited data have suggested transcatheter mitral valve intervention as an alternative treatment in patients at high surgical risk; this may be feasible in the acute setting. MS with CS is not a rare situation worldwide and affects younger patients more than the other VHDs. Urgent BMV appears feasible in critically ill patients, even pregnant patients, and may be considered as the first-line therapy.[4]

Greater results with BMV are seen in individuals with a Wilkins echocardiographic score of 8 or lower, a crisp opening snap, and no calcium in the commissures. The presence of an opening snap confirms the mobility and pliability of the mitral valve, as the snap disappears and the first heart sound amplitude decreases when the mitral valve becomes severely calcified and immobilized. Appropriate candidate selection is a critical step when predicting the immediate results of BMW, and assessment of the anatomy of the mitral valve is essential to eliminate contraindications and define prognostic considerations. The main contraindication for this technique is the presence of an LA thrombus and the performance of TEE before the procedure is required.[12]

The mechanism of successful BMV is splitting of the fused commissures toward the mitral annulus, resulting in the widening of the commissure. In addition, in patients with calcific MS, the balloons could increase mitral valve flexibility by fracture of the calcified deposits in the mitral valve leaflets. Although rare, undesirable complications include leaflets tears; tear of the atrial septum; LV perforation leading to hemopericardium; rupture of chordae, mitral annulus, and papillary muscle; and severe MR, causing hemodynamic collapse or refractory pulmonary edema.[12]

■ AORTIC VALVE DISEASE AND TRANSCATHETER INTERVENTION

Aortic Stenosis

Aortic stenosis (AS) is the most frequent valve disease leading to surgery or transcatheter intervention in developed countries. CS related to AS is a dramatic scenario, with a short-term mortality rate of up to 70% without durable intervention. As current guidelines for AS with CS are very elusive, and a clear-cut strategy cannot yet be defined, and therapeutic interventions in this scenario remain challenging due to the paucity of available data. Whereas medical treatment alone is an unreliable option and surgery is often deemed prohibitive, it is unclear whether direct TAVR or balloon aortic valvuloplasty (BAV) followed by elective TAVR after medical stabilization should be performed, which highlights the strong need for a dedicated large randomized trial that can shed more light on the issue for optimal clinical decision making in this extremely high-risk group of patients.[4]

Indications

Indications for aortic valve replacement (surgical or transcatheter) are as follows:

- Severe high-gradient AS with symptoms (class I recommendation, level B evidence)
- Asymptomatic patients with severe AS and LVEF less than 50% (class I recommendation, level B evidence)
- Severe AS when undergoing other cardiac surgery (class I recommendation, level B evidence)
- Asymptomatic severe AS and low surgical risk (class IIa recommendation, level B evidence)
- Symptomatic with low-flow/low-gradient severe AS (class IIa recommendation, level B evidence)
- Moderate AS and undergoing other cardiac surgery (class IIa recommendation, level C evidence)

TAVR is approved for the following:

- Low to prohibitive surgical risk patients with severe AS
- Valve-in-valve procedures for failed prior bioprosthetic valves

Contraindications

- Absence of a heart team and no cardiac surgery on site
- Estimated life expectancy less than 1 year
- Comorbidity suggesting lack of improvement of quality of life
- Inadequate annulus size (<18 mm, >29 mm)

- Symmetric valve calcification
- Short distance between the annulus and the coronary ostium
- Plaques with mobile thrombi in the ascending aorta
- Hemodynamic instability, LVEF less than 20%, severe pulmonary hypertension with right ventricular dysfunction
- Echocardiographic evidence of intracardiac mass, thrombus, or vegetation
- Hypertrophic cardiomyopathy
- Mixed aortic valve disease (concomitant aortic regurgitation) or significant aortic disease
- Severe MR
- MI within the last 30 days
- MRI confirmed cerebrovascular accident or transient ischemic attack (TIA) within past 6 months
- Inadequate vascular access for transfemoral or subclavian approach (such patients could be treated from the transapical approach)
- Congenital unicuspid or bicuspid valve (no longer applicable)
- End-stage renal disease[13]

Transcatheter Aortic Valve Replacement

Since the first transcatheter implantation of an aortic valve in 2002, TAVR has been successfully established as the treatment for patients with severe AS who are at prohibitive or high risk for surgical aortic valve replacement. Moreover, it is emerging as a viable treatment strategy in the urgent/emergency setting for hemodynamically unstable patients; however, data on emergency TAVR are limited. Outcomes have improved over the years, mainly as a result of appropriate patient selection, major technical refinements, and growing operator experience.[14,15]

Aortic THV consists of a 3-leaflet valve, made of bovine or porcine pericardium or polymeric material, mounted on a radiopaque metallic scaffold (frame), made of stainless steel, nitinol, or cobalt-chromium, and wrapped by an outer sheath (skirt or wrap)—in pericardial or polymeric material—to increase the surface area contact between the device and the native valve, mitigating the risk of significant PVL. According to the position of the prosthetic leaflets relative to the native valve annulus, the THV is labeled as supra- or intra-annular. Supra-annular valves usually result in a larger effective orifice area (EOA) and lower transvalvular aortic mean gradients than intra-annular THVs, which have a lower frame height that eases coronary access.[16]

Some THVs can be recaptured and repositioned after implantation, whereas other THVs are nonrepositionable after deployment. The delivery systems differ regarding the degree of flexion of the distal catheter and sheath diameter. The most common delivery approach is transfemoral, but other access routes (ie, transsubclavian, transaortic, transapical, transcarotid, and transcaval) are also used, as iliofemoral and aortic vessel diseases are frequently present in TAVR patients.[16]

Aortic valve prostheses can be divided into early- and new-generation valves according to their development timeline. Early-generation transcatheter aortic valves mainly comprised the CoreValve (Medtronic, Minneapolis, Minnesota) and the SAPIEN/SAPIEN XT (Edwards Lifesciences, Irvine, California) valves. These valves usually include a relatively large delivery system profile, with no retrievable function or antileakage design. The new-generation transcatheter aortic valves have been developed with improvements in antileakage design such as an outer skirt, retrievable function, and a low delivery system profile. Depending on different valve expansion mechanisms, prostheses are generally divided into balloon-expandable (BE), self-expanding valve (SE), and mechanical expandable (ME). Comparisons among different TAVR devices are still limited, and the choice of a specific prosthesis depends on various factors, such as annulus dimension, distribution of calcium, peripheral vasculature, coronary ostium height, and single operator preferences or center expertise.[1,16,17] (See Table 2-4 and Figure 2-6.)

Balloon-Expandable Valves (BE-THV)

These valves will require a balloon inflation for their expansion under rapid ventricular pacing, which is not always well tolerated in patients with reduced LV systolic function or renal dysfunction. All BE-THVs are intra-annular, are not repositionable, and have a lower stent frame profile, which facilitates coronary access as compared to the SE-THV group. Furthermore, the delivery system allows for greater steerability than SE- or ME-THV, helping in the valve implantation in these patients with complex vascular anatomy, such as in case of horizontal aorta, defined as an aortic angulation of greater than 60 degrees. The first THV implanted (Cribier-Edwards) SAPIEN devices (Edwards Lifesciences) and the Myval THV (Meril Life Sciences, Gujarat, India) are from the BE-THV group. The SAPIEN 3 and SAPIEN 3 Ultra are FDA approved. The SAPIEN 3 consists of a trileaflet bovine pericardial valve mounted in a cobalt-chromium frame with an outer seal cuff to decrease any PVL; in the SAPIEN 3 Ultra,

■ TABLE 2-4. Overview of Transcatheter Aortic Valve Replacement (TAVR) Prostheses

Prosthesis	Frame Material	Leaflet Material	Valve Sizes (mm)	Sheath Sizes	Supra- or Intra-Annular	Repositionable/ Retrievable	Delivery Routes	FDA Approval	CE Mark Approval
Balloon-expandable									
Sapien	Stainless steel	Bovine pericardium	23, 26	22F (23 mm), 24F (26 mm)	Intra-annular	No/No	TF, TA	√	√
Sapien XT	Cobalt-chromium	Bovine pericardium	23, 26, 29	16F (23 mm), 18F (26 mm), 20F (29 mm)	Intra-annular	No/No	TF, TA, TAo	√	√
Sapien 3	Cobalt-chromium	Bovine pericardium	20, 23, 26, 29	14F (20, 23, 26 mm), 16F (29 mm)	Intra-annular	No/No	TF, TA, Tao	√	√
Sapien 3 Ultra	Cobalt-chromium	Bovine pericardium	20, 23, 26, 29	14F	Intra-annular	No/No	TF	√	√
Myval THV	Nickel-cobalt	Bovine pericardium	20, 23, 26, 29, 21.5, 24.5, 27.5, 30.5, 32	14F	Intra-annular	No/No	TF		√
Self-expanding									
CoreValve	Nitinol	Porcine pericardium	23, 26, 29, 31	18F	Supra-annular	Yes/Yes	TF, TAo, SC	√	√
Evolut R	Nitinol	Porcine pericardium	23, 26, 29, 34	14F (23, 26, 29 mm), 16F (34 mm)	Supra-annular	Yes/Yes	TF, TAo, SC	√	√
Evolut PRO	Nitinol	Porcine pericardium	23, 26, 29, 34	16F	Supra-annular	Yes/Yes	TF, TAo, SC	√	√
Evolut PRO+	Nitinol	Porcine pericardium	23, 26, 29, 34	14F (23, 26, 29 mm), 16F (34 mm)	Supra-annular	Yes/Yes	TF, TAo, SC	√	√
ACURATE neo	Nitinol	Porcine pericardium	23, 25, 27	18F	Supra-annular	No/No	TF, TA		√
ACURATE neo2	Nitinol	Porcine pericardium	23, 25, 27	14F	Supra-annular	No/No	TF, TA		√
Allegra	Nitinol	Bovine pericardium	23, 27, 31	18F	Supra-annular	Yes/Yes	TF		

								CE Mark	FDA Approval
Hydra	Nitinol	Bovine pericardium	22, 26, 30	18F	Supra-annular	Yes/Yes	TF		√
Engager	Nitinol	Bovine pericardium	23, 26	30F	Supra-annular	Yes/Yes	TA		√
Venus-A valve	Nitinol	Porcine pericardium	23, 26, 29, 32		Supra-annular	Yes/No	TF		
VitaFlow	Nitinol	Bovine pericardium	21, 24, 27, 30	16F (21, 24 mm), 18F (27, 30 mm)	Supra-annular	Yes/No	TF, TAo, CA		√
VitaFlow Liberty	Nitinol	Bovine pericardium	21, 24, 27, 30	16F (21, 24 mm), 18F (27, 30 mm)	Supra-annular	Yes/No	TF, TAo, CA		√
Centera	Nitinol	Bovine pericardium	23, 26 29	14F	Intra-annular	Yes/Yes	TF		√
Portico	Nitinol	Bovine pericardium	23, 25, 27, 29	18F (23, 25 mm), 19F (27, 29 mm)	Intra-annular	Yes/Yes	TF, TAo, TAx, SC		√
Navitor	Nitinol	Bovine pericardium	23, 25, 27, 29	14F (23, 25 mm), 15F (27, 29 mm)	Intra-annular	Yes/Yes	TF, TAo, Tax		√
Mechanically expandable									
Lotus	Nitinol	Bovine pericardium	23, 25, 27	20F (23, 25 mm), 22F (27 mm)	Intra-annular	Yes/Yes	TF, TAo	√	√
Lotus Edge	Nitinol	Bovine pericardium	23, 25, 27	15F	Intra-annular	Yes/Yes	TF, TAo	√	√
Lotus Mantra	Nitinol	Bovine pericardium	23, 25, 27	12F	Intra-annular	Yes/Yes	TF, TAo	√	√
Aortic regurgitation									
JenaValve	Nitinol	Porcine pericardium	23, 25, 27	19F	Intra-annular	Yes/Yes	TA		√
J-Valve	Nitinol	Bovine pericardium	22, 25, 28	18F	Intra-annular	No/No	TA		√

√ = approved; CA, carotid; CE Mark Approval, approved for use across all European Union member states, European economic area, and Turkey by the European Commission; FDA Approval, approved for use by the United States Food and Drug Administration; SC, subclavian; TA, transapical; TAo, transaortic; TAx, transaxillary; TF, transfemoral.

Source: Reproduced from Chiarito M, et al. Evolving Devices and Material in Transcatheter Aortic Valve Replacement: What to Use and for Whom. *J Clin Med.* 2022; 11: 4445.

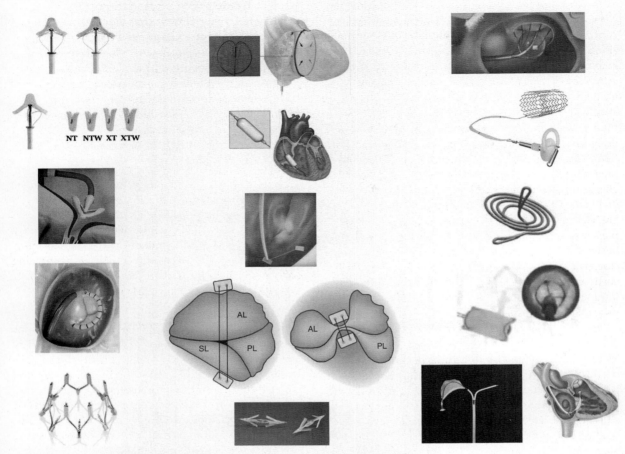

FIGURE 2-6. Current devices for transcatheter tricuspid valve repair. (See color insert.)

the frame height was increased to achieve further rate reduction for PVL. Myval THV consists of a nickel-cobalt alloy (MP35N) frame, a trileaflet valve of bovine pericardium tissue, and an external polymeric sealing cuff. It acquired a CE mark in 2019, but FDA approval is still pending.[1,16]

Self-Expanding Valves (SE-THV)

The SE valves are designed to anchor by progressively being released and, unlike BE-THV, do not require balloon assistance during their deployment.[1] The majority of SE-THVs are supra-annular, which results in a higher EOA, lower gradients, and lower possibility for severe prosthesis-patient mismatch (PPM). Moreover, it is not mandatory to perform rapid ventricular pacing during implantation, and most SE-THVs may be repositionable and/or retrievable, at the expense of limited steerability.

The first SE-THV developed was the Medtronic CoreValve (Medtronic, Sunnyvale, CA), and along with all its subsequent generations (Evolut R, Evolut PRO, and Evolut PRO+), they represent the most studied and commonly implanted SE-THVs achieving CE and FDA approval. The Evolut PRO+ added an outer porcine pericardial tissue wrap that increases surface area contact and tissue interaction between the THV and the native aortic annulus. The greater frame height of SE-THV can make access to coronaries more challenging, and because of its higher radial force, higher pressures are exerted on the membranous septum and on the conduction system compared to BE-THV, causing a considerable risk of conduction disorders requiring pacemaker implantation. The ACURATE neo (older generation) and ACURATE neo2 (newer generation), produced by Boston Scientific, differ from the Evolut

THV by having a top-down deployment, which can control the implant depth; in addition, it is nonrepositionable and predilation of the aortic valve is strongly recommended.

Among SE-THVs, some are intra-annular, such as Centera (Edwards), Portico (Abbott Structural Heart, Westfield, IN), and its iteration Navitor (Abbott Structural Heart). The Portico valve has a leaflet geometry designed to function in an elliptical or round configuration. This valve is also self-expanding, retrievable, and fully resheathable. The annular positioning facilitates the engagement of coronary ostia after implantation. It is CE and FDA (September 2021) approved. The Navitor THV has been designed with an active outer fabric cuff, which is the key to decrease the PVL. SE-THV with supra-annular designs are particularly indicated in patients with a severely calcified and small annulus and TAVR-in-surgical aortic valve replacement (SAVR), and both supra- and intra-annular valves are indicated in patients at risk for poor tolerance to rapid pacing.

Other SE-THVs with CE but not FDA approval are the following: Hydra (Vascular Innovations Co., Nonthaburi, Thailand), the mechanism of which consists of recapturing during release; Allegra (NVT AG, Muri, Switzerland); whose grip uses a "squeeze-to-release" mechanism that prevents undesired rotation during the implantation; and Engager (Medtronic) and Venus-A valve (Venus Medtech, Hangzhou, China). VitaFlow (Microport, Shanghai, China) and its subsequent iteration VitaFlow Liberty are novel THVs manufactured in China with ongoing approval for CE mark.[16]

Complications of TAVR

Paravalvular regurgitation (PVR). PVR has been associated with poor survival after BE-TAVR. With newer generation valves, there is a slightly lower rate of PVR (mild 40% and moderate to severe 2%-8%) compared to older generations (40% mild PVR and 10% more than mild). This can be attributed to the increasing use of CT imaging for preprocedure sizing, as well as the development of external adaptive skirts on newer devices. Compared to the SAPIEN XT, the SAPIEN 3 has been associated with a much lower rate of moderate or severe PVR (3.5%) and reduced need for balloon after dilatation.

Conduction disturbances. This is a frequent complication of TAVR, with an incidence for new PPM implant of 8.8% of patients undergoing TAVR (with SAPIEN)

based on the PARTNER trial and in its continued access registry. A lower implanted valve has been associated with new bundle branch block, complete heart block, and PPM need. Furthermore, in this registry, some predictors of permanent pacemaker implantation included right bundle branch block, prosthesis diameter/LV outflow tract diameter (for each 0.1 increment), LV end-diastolic diameter (for each 1 cm), and treatment in the continued access registry).

Malpositioning. This is a largely preventable complication; however, it can be associated with early operator experience as well as use of a first-generation device, as these were known to move cranially during inflation. An improved understanding of the procedure would likely minimize this possibility and mitigate the consequences should malposition occur, as subvalvular positioning may result in severe aortic regurgitation due to lack of seal at the annulus with the skirt of the prosthesis.

Aortic root/annular rupture. This is a major life-threatening concern with BE TAVR, and the risk for rupture has been associated with heavy LV outflow tract calcification (nearly 11-fold higher risk of rupture), aggressive 2% or greater annular area oversizing (8- to 9-fold higher risk of rupture), and postdilatation. The incidence of severe oversizing may be reduced with a multislice CT-based assessment of aortic annulus dimension in conjunction with adapted sizing guidelines for preprocedure planning.

Bleeding and vascular complications. Unfortunately, the risk for any bleeding after TAVR is as high as approximately 30% and is independently associated with a nearly 3-fold higher risk of 1-year mortality (hazard ratio [HR], 2.54; 95% confidence interval [CI], 1.3-4.9; $P = .002$). Earlier studies involving the SAPIEN THV showed an approximate 20% rate of vascular complications, including dissection (necessitating stenting) and perforations/rupture (requiring surgical bypass). This risk decreases with improved operator experience and reduced size of the delivery catheter sheaths. The incidence of vascular complications with current-generation SAPIEN XT and SAPIEN 3 systems is approximately 5%.

Stroke. Major safety concerns were raised from previous randomized studies showing increased stroke/TIA rates with TAVR compared to medical treatment and SAVR. A recent meta-analysis of over 10,000 patients undergoing transfemoral (TF) or transapical or transsubclavian TAVR for native severe AS showed an overall

30-day stroke/TIA risk of 3.3% (range, 0%-6%), with the majority being major strokes (2.9%). The incidence increased up to 5.2% during the first year after TAVR. Depending on the approach and prosthetic valve use, the rate for this complication varied, with the lowest rate after the transapical approach with the SAPIEN THV (2.7%). Compared to patients without stroke, patients with stroke had a nearly 4-fold higher 30-day mortality (25.5% vs 6.9%). Recent data utilizing the SAPIEN 3 device demonstrated significantly lower stroke rates in high- and intermediate-risk patients (any stroke ~2.5%, major stroke ~1%). Although reduction in the number of new lesions has been demonstrated with cerebral embolic protection filters, larger studies are currently in progress to assess the impact of cerebral embolic protection filters on neuroimaging and neurologic symptoms.[15,18,19]

Transcatheter Valve-in-Valve Intervention

This procedure is performed by implanting a THV within a failing bioprosthetic valve. In comparison with a reoperative SAVR, the transcatheter valve-in-valve (ViV) operation is a less invasive procedure; however, it has been associated with specific complications. Therefore, it requires extensive preoperative evaluation and planning by the heart team.[1] The heterogeneity of each bioprosthetic valve size and type, mode of failure (calcification vs leaflet tear, tissue valve stenosis vs regurgitation), valve position (aortic, mitral, tricuspid, pulmonary), type of THV implanted, delivery system access, and depth of implant can all dramatically alter the procedural success and outcomes.

The safety and feasibility of the transcatheter ViV implantation were demonstrated in an international multicenter registry for patients with surgical bioprosthetic valve deterioration. Furthermore, the 2020 American College of Cardiology (ACC)/American Heart Association (AHA) guidelines and 2017 European Society of Cardiology/European Association for Cardiothoracic Surgery guidelines for VHD management stated that transcatheter ViV implantation is a reasonable alternative to reoperation in surgical high-risk patients or those who are unable to undergo surgery with surgical bioprosthetic failure and limited valve expansion because of inability to use original surgical prostheses, leading to a risk of PPM.[1] The transcatheter ViV has been approved by the FDA for use in the aortic position for both the CoreValve and SAPIEN XT valves since 2015. The complications that have been related to ViV procedures are coronary

obstruction and malposition, high postprocedural gradients, and possible migration of the valve.[33]

Percutaneous Balloon Aortic Valvuloplasty

Percutaneous BAV (PBAV) was first described by Alain Cribier in 1986 to treat patients with severe AS. Unfavorable midterm outcomes related to early restenosis have rapidly limited its indications. However, in patients with AS and CS, PBAV was shown to be lifesaving in some circumstances. Since transcatheter aortic valve implantation (TAVI) was developed, BAV has been considered with a renewed interest as part of the procedure and may be indicated as a bridge to further interventions in very high-risk patients. Survivors may be bridged to TAVI or SAVR or treated medically according to the heart team judgment. The decision should be made considering the life expectancy related to age, general status, comorbidities, and operative risk.[20]

Contraindications for PBAV include moderate to severe aortic regurgitation (AR), endocarditis, an intracardiac mass, active infection, and the presence of a contraindication to antithrombolytic therapy in the perioperative setting. Early studies reported high complication rates of up to 25%, with vascular complications being the frequent complication. Other complications reported at varying rates include periprocedural MI, development or worsening of AR, stroke, systemic embolization, conduction abnormalities, ventricular perforation, cardiac tamponade, and death.[21]

■ AORTIC REGURGITATION

Although TAVR has been adopted as a mainstay therapy for AS, SAVR continues to be the gold standard therapy for patients with symptomatic severe AR/aortic insufficiency (AI). Unfortunately, because of their excessive surgical risk, many patients with severe AI cannot undergo surgical intervention. Current US FDA-approved TAVR prostheses rely on calcification of the native aortic valve to anchor the prosthesis in place. Although TAVR devices have been used off-label to treat selected patients with AI, these TAVR devices cannot be reliably implanted in the native valve AI annuli due to challenges with the placement and anchoring of the device. Thus, it is not surprising that the outcomes with TAVR in patients with pure AI are worse in comparison with patients with AS, with some complications including inadequate valve sealing with significant PVL and valve embolization. Although some operators choose TAVR for AI, they frequently rely on oversizing TAVR device techniques to improve valve anchoring. Self-expanding THVs have been preferred for cases with pure native valve AI because of their ability to oversize the valve prosthesis by relying on the radial force of the valve while minimizing the risk of annular rupture.[22]

A first-generation device designed for transapical implantation was evaluated in the JUPITER (JenaValve Evaluation of Long Term Performance and Safety in Patients With Severe Aortic Stenosis of Aortic Insufficiency) registry. In a series of 31 patients, the procedural success was 96.7%, and all-cause mortality was 10% at 1-year follow-up. This device is currently under investigation in the ALIGN-AR study (JenaValve Pericardial TAVR Aortic Regurgitation Study).[22]

The JenaValve (JenaValve Technology, München, Germany), a porcine pericardial valve in a low-profile nitinol frame with a paper clip–like fixation mechanism, is currently the only THV with a CE mark for use in patients with AR. The J-Valve (JC Medical, New York, New York) is another device that can be used for the treatment of native AR, as well as AS, and is currently being studied in an early feasibility study in the United States. Two further valves from China, the Venus-AVR valve (Venus Medtech) and VitaFlowVR (Microport), are at an advanced stage of development with high rates of procedural success in the challenging cohort of patients with a bicuspid aortic valve (Figure 2-6).[16]

■ TRICUSPID VALVE DISEASE AND TRANSCATHETER INTERVENTION

Tricuspid valve (TV) regurgitation and stenosis are rare VHDs, and they both can be treated medically; however, they often require more invasive interventions such as surgical repair of the valve. Percutaneous intervention, or transcatheter valve repair, has become a more popular method than surgery in recent years, especially in nonsurgical candidates. Additionally, percutaneous intervention on the aortic and mitral valves has helped the search for more percutaneous approaches to repair other cardiac valves over the past several years.[23]

Unlike established mitral and aortic transcatheter valve intervention criteria, currently, the only established criteria for tricuspid procedural therapy for severe tricuspid disease are limited to surgical valve repair or replacement for primary TV disease with presenting symptoms of right-sided HF or for patients who are already planned to undergo

cardiac surgery. Unfortunately, this approach can delay procedural-based therapies to late stages in the natural history of the disease process. Thus, medical therapy, timing of treatment, types of intervention (repair vs replacement), and clinical outcomes remain a challenge in designing clinical trials and evaluating the success of transcatheter therapies.[24]

Indications

- Severe tricuspid stenosis with associated symptoms (gradient >5 cm or surface area <1 cm)
- Severe symptomatic primary or secondary tricuspid regurgitation
- Patient undergoing left-sided valve surgery with moderate to severe primary tricuspid regurgitation or tricuspid stenosis (symptomatic or asymptomatic) or mild to moderate progressive functional (secondary) tricuspid regurgitation with a dilated annulus (>40 mm or >21 mm/m^2)
- TV endocarditis
- Asymptomatic or mildly symptomatic primary tricuspid regurgitation with progressive right ventricular dilatation and/or dysfunction
- Carcinoid involvement of the TV
- Congenital malformations of the TV
- Traumatic or iatrogenic injuries to the valve (pacemaker wires or during heart or lung biopsy)
- Undergoing other cardiac procedures with tricuspid disease

Contraindications

- Thrombus in the femoral, jugular, right atrium, or the superior/inferior vena cava
- Good surgical candidate who would benefit more from an open repair
- Unable to tolerate systemic anticoagulation or bleeding disorder with coagulopathy[23]

Tricuspid Regurgitation

The etiology of TV regurgitation (TR) can be divided into primary and secondary/functional tricuspid disease. Primary TV disease accounts for only 10% to 20% of cases of severe TR, with secondary/functional tricuspid disease accounting for the majority of cases.

Primary TV pathology includes congenital heart disease (Ebstein anomaly, TV dysplasia, leaflet tethering from perimembranous ventricular septal defect, atrioventricular septal defects with "cleft" leaflets), myxomatous valve disease, and acquired medical and structural valve disease processes (endocarditis, rheumatic, carcinoid, radiation or drug induced, leaflet tear/prolapse, chordal rupture, right ventricular [RV] pacing/defibrillator leads, intravascular trauma from procedures, chest wall trauma). Secondary TR occurs mainly from dilation of the annulus andenlargement of the RV secondary to left-sided heart disease (LV dysfunction and mitral valve disease), RV volume and pressure overload, and dilation of cardiac chambers from pulmonary arterial disease with pulmonary hypertension (primary pulmonary arterial disease, chronic lung disease, thromboembolic disease), acquired RV dysfunction (RV myocardial disease, RV ischemia/infarction), and atrial fibrillation.[24,25]

Despite that the prevalence of moderate-to-severe TR in the United States exceeds 1.6 million and is associated with a 1-year mortality rate of 20% to 40%, therapy often includes observation or diuretics in the setting of right-sided HF, and surgical intervention is rare, with only 8000 TV operations performed annually in the United States. There are some transcatheter-based therapies for valvular disease now available for treatment of TR; however, most procedures are performed in the setting of clinical trials or off-label use.[24]

Transcatheter TV repair (TTVR) technologies are based on reproducing surgical concepts such as annuloplasty or leaflet adoption, but also alternative approaches are under investigation such as coaptation enhancement or heterotopic caval valve implantation.[26] TTVR can be classified according to the mechanism of action as follows: annuloplasty devices and coaptation devices (spacer and edge-to-edge leaflet repair). (See Figure 2-7.)

Coaptation Devices

MitraClip, TriClip, and Other Devices The TRILUMINATE (Trial to Evaluate Treatment With Abbott Transcatheter Clip Repair System in Patients With Moderate or Greater TR) trial assessed a dedicated TEER system with the first-generation TriClip system for treatment of the TR by clamping via the femoral vein, the anterior and septal leaflet, or the posterior and septal leaflet, similar to Mitra-Clip. At 1 year, 87% of the patients had 1 grade reduction in TR, clinical improvement in NYHA class I/II to 83% from a baseline of 31%, and improvement in the Kansas City Cardiomyopathy Questionnaire (KCCQ) by 20 ± 2.61 points. The TriClip system became the first approved transcatheter TV repair device in the world by achieving the CE mark in April 2020.[1,26] Notably, the new MitraClip G4 system and TriClip G4 system now have independent leaflet grasping arms that were not available during the TRILUMINATE trial.

The MitraClip system consists of 2 clips arms made of cobalt-chromium and covered in polyester and the delivery system. In the international multimeter registry data from the international TriValve registry (Transcatheter TV Therapies), the MitraClip device was the most used device (66% of the cases) for severe TR or combined TMVR and TTVR. The 2 common techniques of using MitraClip for TR are (1) the triple-orifice technique, where 2 clips are applied between the septal-anterior and septal-posterior leaflets to convert TV opening into 3 orifices; and (2) the bicuspidalization technique, where 2 clips are applied between the anterior and septal leaflets.

PASCAL System The PASCAL device (Edwards Lifesciences) consists of a 22-F delivery catheter and the nitinol-based device with a 10-mm spacer and contoured broad paddles for leaflet grasping. It was also employed for patients with MR, and a single-arm, US-based, early feasibility study for the Edwards PASCAL (Edwards PASCAL Transcatheter Valve Repair System in Tricuspid Regurgitation [CLASP TR]) suggested that this device has high procedural success and acceptable safety, with significant clinical improvement. Currently, the ongoing pivotal clinical CLASP II TR trial for safety and effectiveness of the PASCAL device for TR is enrolling patients.

The FORMA Device The FORMA device (Edwards Lifesciences) was designed to occupy the regurgitant orifice while providing a surface for coaptation. It consists of a spacer and a rail that is anchored to the RV apex. The spacer is a polymer-filled balloon that expands via the holes in the spacer shaft and is positioned fluoroscopically, via left subclavian or axillary vein. Long-term outcomes with the FORMA device showed a marked reduction in severe TR from 95% to 33% at 2-year follow-up, along with a significant increase in quality-of-life markers including NYHA class, KCCQ scores, and 6-minute walk distance. In addition, there was significant reduction in peripheral edema. No complications related to the device or vascular access were observed during follow-up. The early feasibility study of this device is currently ongoing and will require further evaluation if its safety. However, this device is only suitable for patients with small regurgitant orifices.[1,24,26]

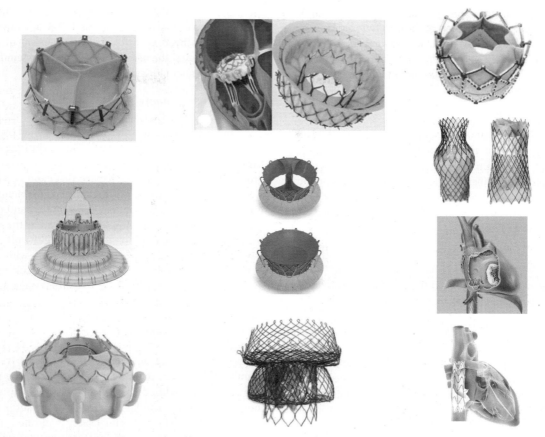

FIGURE 2-7. Transcatheter tricuspid valve replacement. (See color insert.)

Emerging Leaflet Coaptation Devices

The Mistral TVRS (Mitralix, Tel Aviv, Israel) is a spiral-shaped nitinol wire device. It grasps the chords from 2 adjacent leaflets and approximates chords and leaflets together. The Mistral device is delivered via an exclusive 7.5-F Mistral delivery system catheter and another off-the-shelf, 8.5-F steerable catheter (Agilis NxT; Abbott Vascular). Currently, the ongoing MATTERS (Mistral Percutaneous Tricuspid Valve Repair FIM) study aims to enroll 20 patients with severe TR in open-label fashion to assess the safety and performance of the Mistral device.

Cerclage-TR block is being refined with funding from the National Institutes of Health (NIH) to implant a leaflet extension at the septal location of the TV. The concept is based on the Mitral Loop Cerclage Annuloplasty device (Tau-PNU Medical, Pusan, South Korea), which has been reported to reduce MR in 4 of 5 patients in FIM study.

The procedure involves placing the device anchor in the subclavian vein and creating a 360-degree loop around the mitral annulus in the pericardium. One arm of the device enters the coronary sinus and septal vein and then perforates the interventricular septum to enter the RV outflow tract (RVOT). From the RVOT, it is snared and externalized via the femoral vein. Subsequently, the second arm of the device enters through the right atrium and is placed underneath the septal tricuspid leaflet. This concept could offer an advantage for patients with concomitant severe MR and TR to treat both valvular diseases simultaneously.

The CroíValve DUO™ Tricuspid Coaptation Valve System was designed to assist coaptation in the dilated tricuspid annulus. It combines the repair and replacement approaches via 2 integrated systems. First, it uses a coaptation valve composed of pericardial tissue as well as a prosthetic valve that works in conjunction with the native valve. Second, an anchor system in the superior vena cava (SVC) secures the position of the coaptation valve using a stent in the SVC. In the initial temporary proof-of-concept early clinical data of 5 patients with massive or torrential TR, TR was reduced to mild among all patients without any adverse events.[24]

Annuloplasty

The tricuspid annuloplasty devices can be classified into 3 main types: direct ring annuloplasty (Cardioband, IRIS), indirect ring annuloplasty (transatrial intrapericardial tricuspid annuloplasty [TRIAPTA] devices), and direct suture annuloplasty (Trialign, minimally invasive annuloplasty [MIA], and pledget-assisted suture tricuspid annuloplasty [PASTA]).

Direct Ring Annuloplasty

Cardioband The Cardioband repair system (Edwards Lifesciences) is an approved therapy for secondary (functional) MR, and studies are currently investigating its use in patients with severe tricuspid regurgitation caused by a dilatation of the right annulus. The Cardioband system is a catheter-based device that functions as a percutaneous annuloplasty band using a transfemoral approach, and its implantation is performed by stainless steel anchors (6 mm long). After cinching of the Cardioband, the device reduces the tricuspid annular dimensions.[26] In April 2018, the Cardioband device received CE mark approval, based on results of the Tricuspid Regurgitation Repair With Cardioband Transcatheter System (TRI-REPAIR) study, which demonstrated a significant improvement in clinical function and echocardiographic outcomes at 6 months and 2 years of follow-up. The Transcatheter Repair of TR With Edwards Cardioband TR System Post Market Study (TriB-AND) is a multicenter, prospective, single-arm, postmarket study that aims to evaluate the safety and effectiveness of the of the Cardioband Tricuspid Reconstruction System.[27]

IRIS Millipede Ring

The IRIS transcatheter annuloplasty ring (Millipede, Santa Rosa, California) is a complete semirigid ring that is placed in the supra-annular position and then anchored and cinched, thereby reducing the TR and annular size. The IRIS implant consists of 3 components: a frame that is made of nitinol formed into a ring, anchors that engage the annular tissue, and collars that reduce the diameter of the frame to achieve a proper valve leaflet coaptation. The IRIS has 2 distinct advantages: first, the ring can be completely adjusted and repositioned before the final deployment, and second,

the ring preserves the native anatomy without precluding future transcatheter options such as TEER. Although this technique has been used for the management of mitral valve pathologies, the use of the Millipede system for TR is currently under clinical development.[27,28]

Indirect Annuloplasty

TRAIPTA TRAIPTA is a concept where, after establishing venous access, pericardial access is obtained by puncturing the right atrial appendage. This technique allows the delivery of an implant along the atrioventricular groove within the pericardial space that exerts compressive forces over the annulus. Interactive adjustment of the implant controls its tension and helps modify and reduce the TR. The right atrial puncture is sealed at the end of the procedure with a nitinol device. While the procedure has been performed in pigs, human testing with a new device is under development. Limitations of such a procedure include the need for a free pericardial space and the risk of coronary artery compression.[28]

Direct Suture Annuloplasty

Trialign The Trialign device (Mitralign, Tewksbury, Massachusetts) is a transcatheter suture-based tricuspid annuloplasty system that attempts to replicate the results of the current modified Kay procedure, which has shown long-term efficacy similar to that of other surgical TV repair methods. The posterior leaflet is plicated using 2 pledgets that are placed at the anteroposterior and septal posterior commissure and then sutured together using the dedicated plication lock device. A distance of 25 to 28 mm between the 2 pledgets is recommended. In case of suboptimal results, a second pair of pledgets can be implanted to obtain a consistent reduction in annular dimensions.

The safety and efficacy of the Trialign system were assessed in the prospective single-arm, open-label, multicenter SCOUT (Percutaneous TV Annuloplasty System [PTVAS] for Symptomatic Chronic Functional TR) trial. This trial enrolled 25 patients with moderate or greater TR and NYHA class greater than II. The primary performance and safety endpoint was procedural success at 30 days. The technical success was 80% with significant echocardiographic reduction in the tricuspid annulus size and EROA. There was a consistent improvement in the quality-of-life metrics, with improvement in NYHA functional class and 6-minute walk test results. Currently, the Safety and Performance of the Trialign PTVAS (SCOUT-II) study aims to enroll 60 participants with symptomatic functional TR from 15 sites in the United States and Europe.[24,26]

PASTA PASTA is a novel experimental transcatheter technique to create a double-orifice TV and is based on the Hetzer's double-orifice suture technique. In PASTA, pledgeted sutures are delivered via a transcatheter approach to oppose septal and lateral targets on the tricuspid annulus, thereby reducing the TV orifice. In a preclinical animal study, PASTA successfully reduced annular and chamber dimensions and TR.[28,29]

MIA The MIA device (Micro Interventional Devices, Newtown, Pennsylvania) was created to replicate surgical annuloplasty for reducing the parameter of tricuspid annulus, thus decreasing the TR. It is a compliant, self-tensioning implant incorporating the company's proprietary PolyCor anchors and MyoLast thermoplastic elastomer that reduces tricuspid annular dimension without direct sutures. MIA tricuspid delivery system consists of a 12-F delivery catheter, PolyCor anchors, and the proprietary suture lock that helps in cinching the tricuspid annulus together to reduce the annular diameter. Initial data from the first 31 patients in the Study of Transcatheter Tricuspid Annular Repair (STTAR) trial demonstrated consistent reduction in the TR grade, EROA, TR vena contracta, and TV diameter at 1 and 6 months. The device is approved by the FDA breakthrough device designation and still pending a CE mark approval.[24,27]

DaVingi TR System The DaVingi TR system (Cardiac Implants, Wilmington, Deleware) is a transcatheter device designed to deliver an annuloplasty ring on the atrial side of the TV using right heart catheterization through the right internal jugular vein. The annuloplasty ring is a small multielement ring, consisting of an outer fabric layer, a preset stakes array, and an internal adjustment cord that can be adjusted at a later stage after the outer layer of the ring and stakes are encapsulated in new tissue growth. The safety and performance of the system will be evaluated in 15 patients with severe TR in the first-in-human study to assess safety and performance of the DaVingi TR system in the management of patients with functional TR.[27]

TriCinch The TriCinch System (4TECH Cardio, Galway, Ireland) is a transcatheter tricuspid annuloplasty device employed to reduce the annulus size using an anchored coil at the junction of the anterior-posterior TV leaflets. The system consists of a Dacron band connecting both the self-expanding stent and a corkscrew anchor. The annular diameter and regurgitation degree were reduced postoperatively when the system was first applied in 2015, and the quality of life improved at 6 months postoperatively. The second-generation TriCinch Coil system had better stability than the first-generation device and successfully converted severe TR to mild TR postoperatively. Device-related complications include hemopericardium and device dehiscence. The manufacturer of the device is currently not enrolling patients for clinical trials.[1,24,26,27]

Transcatheter Tricuspid Valve Implantation

The 2TV replacement strategies include orthotropic transcatheter valve replacement and heterotopic valve replacement where the aim is to reduce the caval regurgitant flow.

Orthotropic Transcatheter Valve Replacement

The tricuspid annulus is a complex and highly dynamic structure offering little resistance for long-term fixation of orthotopic valves. In patients with severe TR, the annulus is massively dilated with a loss of anatomic landmarks; hence, the development of transcatheter orthotopic valve implantation comes with specific challenges, including device fixation, sizing, paravalvular sealing, and thrombogenicity in a low-flow, low-pressure circulation.

The NaviGate Transcatheter Tricuspid Valve This device has been developed for orthotopic correction of severe functional TR by NaviGate Cardiac Structures (Lake Forest, California). The bioprosthetic self-expanding valve with a size of up to 52 mm has been successfully implanted in compassionate cases using either the jugular vein or atrium approach.[1,26] Thus far, this valve has been employed in high-risk surgical patients with TR in multiple clinical centers. Results have demonstrated that this device has effectively improved cardiac function and right heart remodeling in patients. However, the problems of PVL and its nonretrievable design pose some challenges related to its usage. In the future, the optimal population for this valve and corresponding long-term outcomes should be studied.[1]

The LuX-Valve The LuX-Valve (Jenscare Biotechnology, Ningbo, Zhejiang, China) is a transcatheter TV replacement device developed in China. It consists of bovine pericardial tissue and nitinol stents in addition to a skirt to prevent PVL. The deployment of this valve does not require radial force but is fixed by a special anchoring structure. Of the 12 patients included in the FIM study of this device, only 1 patient died in the hospital due to MI.[1]

EVOQUE Tricuspid Valve Replacement System The EVOQUE system (Edwards Lifesciences) is a nitinol, self-expanding, bioprosthetic valve composed of bovine tissue that is delivered transfemorally via a 28-F system and anchored within the TV. The EVOQUE valve comes in multiple sizes (52, 48, and 44 mm) to address a broad range of tricuspid pathologies and anatomies.[29]

INTREPID System The INTREPID system (Medtronic, Fridley, Minnesota) is a novel, nitinol, self-expanding, bioprosthetic valve composed of bovine tissue that can be delivered via a 35-F venous access point. The valve is available in 3 outer frame sizes (43-, 46-, or 50-mm diameter), with a 27-mm inner stent frame. The INTREPID system differentiates itself from other transcatheter TV systems in that it does not require leaflet capturing for anchoring, but rather is anchored by deploying a large, fluted, atrial brim on the atrial side of the valve. This brim is flexible and conforms to the atrial shape under which the stiffer ventricular portion sits. Theoretically, this should improve implantation success in those with delicate valve anatomy, and, in one case, it was shown to be feasible in the presence of pacing leads. The first-in-human use of INTREPID in tricuspid position has been implemented as compassionate use in the first 3 patients. The TTVR Early Feasibility Study aims to enroll 15 participants with severe TR to undergo TV replacement using the Intrepid TTVR system.[24,29]

Heterotopic Transcatheter Tricuspid Valve Implantation
Heterotopic implantation of a balloon or self-expanding valve in the IVC, cranial to the hepatic veins, has been done in a limited number of end-stage patients, aiming at reducing venous hypertension in the hepatorenal system. Likewise, the addition of a valve in the SVC would prevent transmission of systolic waveforms of right atrial hypertension into the superior central systemic venous system. However, with this approach, the right atrium undergoes a potentially detrimental ventricularization process.[5]

Lauten et al first proposed the idea of prosthesis in the vena cava to reduce TR and relieve HF symptoms.[30] The Edwards SAPIEN XT valve and TricValve (P & F Products & Features Vertriebs GmbH, Vienna, Austria), a self-expanding valve with 2 separate stents, were reported to be first used in humans in 2013 and 2014, respectively. The Edwards SAPIEN XT valve is effective for improving dyspnea but has a high in-hospital mortality rate.[1]

Caval dilation remains the main limitation in both devices, as the IVC may dilate up to 35 mm in diameter, while the SVC may dilate up to 40 mm in chronic severe TR due to volume overload. The tapered dilatation of the SVC makes placement of the SAPIEN valve challenging, which is why the TricValve is preferred in this location. It is currently believed that bicaval caval valve implantation (CAVI) is not superior to implantation in the IVC alone, although this still requires further analysis.[29]

Finally, although the registries presented above have shown excellent procedural success and safety in the short term, device embolization remains a potential complication of this procedure. The TRICAVAL trial, a randomized controlled trial of CAVI with the SAPIEN valve versus optimal medical therapy, had to be terminated early due to 28.5% of patients having device embolization requiring open surgical retrieval. Ongoing clinical trials, including the HOVER trial (Heterotopic Implantation of the Edwards SAPIEN Transcatheter Aortic Valve in the IVC for the Treatment of Severe Tricuspid Regurgitation) with the SAPIEN valve and the TRICUS STUDY Euro (Safety and Efficacy of the TricValve Device) with the TricValve, aim to shed further light on the safety and efficacy of CAVI.[29]

The TriCento bioprosthesis (New Valve Technology, Hechingen, Germany) is a 13.5-cm covered stent with landing zones in the SVC and IVC and a low intra-atrial porcine bicuspid valve segment. There is also a short non-covered segment to allow for hepatic vein outflow. The stent is custom made based on preprocedure imaging. Access is transfemoral via a 24-F sheath. The first-in-human implantation in 2017 reported successful device function and reduced caval vein regurgitant volume after 3 months. Since then, a total of 31 TriCento bioprostheses have been implanted in Europe.[31]

Tricuspid Stenosis

Tricuspid stenosis (TS) is mostly secondary to rheumatic heart disease. Isolated TS is rare as it is usually associated with some form of TR. The pathophysiology of TS is similar to mitral valve stenosis in which the chordae have shortening with fusion and leaflet thickening. Calcific deposits of the valve occur late in the disease process.[23]

Percutaneous transcatheter repair of the TV with stenosis can be performed using double-balloon valvotomy or valvuloplasty. Intervention can be performed on native TV stenosis or on the stenosis of a bioprosthetic valve. There are multiple options for TS intervention. Double-balloon valvotomy is a common treatment for TS, and single-balloon valvuloplasty is another option. Treatment of severe TS includes valve replacement as a first-line option. Percutaneous repair should be reserved for patients who are at high risk for open surgical repair.[23]

Complications of Tricuspid Valve Transcatheter Intervention

The complications associated with TV repair are similar whether intervention is performed via open repair or transcatheter repair. Mortality with TV replacement is 3 to 4 times higher than with other single-valve open or percutaneous procedures. Surgical intervention for tricuspid disease can be associated with a high risk of morbidity and mortality, with perioperative mortality reaching up to 10% in selected cases. Complications include the following:

- MI due to damage or irritation to the right coronary artery
- Arrhythmias and heart blocks
- Catheter-related complications to access site (hematoma, arteriotomy, dissection, arteriovenous fistula)
- Prosthetic valve malfunction
- HF
- Perioperative bleeding and resulting blood product transfusion
- Infection of surgical site and/or the valve prosthesis
- Sepsis
- Pulmonary complications (pneumothorax, pneumonia, embolisms)
- Renal failure (due to concomitant use of contrast dye)
- Stroke[23]

■ PULMONARY VALVE DISEASE AND TRANSCATHETER INTERVENTION

Pulmonary Regurgitation and Stenosis

After congenital heart disease surgery, the RVOT is often subject to pulmonary regurgitation (PR) and/or stenosis (PS), which has been shown to lead to insidious dilation and progressive risk of irreversible systolic dysfunction, arrhythmia, and sudden death.[32]

The earliest transcatheter pulmonary valve replacement/implantation (TPVR/TPVI) technique was performed in 2000; this surgery is mainly performed to treat patients with PR after surgery for complex congenital heart diseases, such as tetralogy of Fallot. Severe PR may cause significantly decreased exercise tolerance and even ventricular arrhythmias or sudden death; therefore, these patients may require surgical valve replacement, which has a high risk of reoperation. TPVI has evolved to become an attractive alternative to surgery in such patients, as supported by the early results of corresponding studies.[1]

Indications

TPVR provides an additional therapeutic option, thereby extending conduit life span and avoiding the need for repeat median sternotomy. The timing for intervention is based on RV volume and function, as well as symptomatology. TPVR is designed for treatment of circumferential RVOT conduit dysfunction when there is evidence of significant PS and/or PR with peak-to-peak gradient of 35 mmHg or greater.[5,32] Indications for TPVR have expanded to its use in patients with pulmonary hypertension, demonstrating the capacity of current valves to function under higher pressures. The off-label use of the Melody valve (Medtronic) for failed bioprosthetic valves in the pulmonary position has also been reported with good safety, efficacy, and short-term durability.[32]

The Melody THV was the first to receive approval. A second TPVR option is now available: the SAPIEN pulmonic THV (Edwards Lifesciences) received the CE mark in 2010 and is currently under investigation in the United States (Figure 2-8).[5]

The Melody THV

The Melody valve received the European CE mark in September 2006, and the first US implant was performed in January 2007. It is used in patients with a clinical indication for intervention and a dysfunctional RVOT conduit or bioprosthetic valve with moderate or greater PR and/or a mean RVOT gradient greater than 35 mmHg. It consists of a bovine jugular vein sutured inside of a platinum iridium stent with currently 2 available valve sizes: the TPV 20 and the TPV 22. Both valves are deployed using the Medtronic Ensemble delivery system, a 22-F delivery system using balloon-in-balloon technology.[33]

SAPIEN Valve

The SAPIEN XT (Edwards Lifesciences) was approved by the FDA in March 2016 for use in dysfunctional RVOT

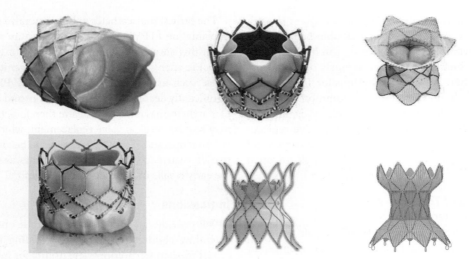

FIGURE 2-8. Transcatheter pulmonary valves. (See color insert.)

conduits using the same criteria as noted for the Melody valve. The SAPIEN XT consists of a trileaflet bovine pericardial valve inside a cobalt-chromium frame and was originally designed for use in the aortic position, as was the Edwards Lifesciences Novaflex delivery system. Compared to the Melody valve, the SAPIEN XT is short, with valve heights varying between 14.3 mm for the 23-mm valve to 19.1 mm for the 29-mm valve.[33]

The SAPIEN S3 is the latest generation of SAPIEN valve, and although it has not yet received FDA approval for implantation in the pulmonary position, it is currently undergoing a clinical trial. There is also increasing experience with off-label use of this valve in centers outside of a clinical trial. Like the XT, the S3 is a trileaflet bovine pericardial valve sewn into a cobalt-chromium stent. However, the S3 has an additional polyethylene terephthalate skirt that is intended to decrease the incidence of PVLs in the aortic position.[33]

Future Directions

Despite the success of using currently available valve technology in patients with native outflow tracts, many patients will nonetheless be unsuitable candidates for this approach. To meet this need, the Medtronic Harmony TPV and the Alterra Adaptive Pre-stent from Edwards Lifesciences were designed and have undergone early clinical trials in the United States. There is insufficient quality evidence in the clinical literature demonstrating the long-term safety and efficacy of the Harmony for TPV.[33]

Complications

Conduit rupture. Conduit rupture is a relatively common adverse event associated with rehabilitation of obstructed conduits and occurs in 19.5% to 22% of patients undergoing angioplasty. Most of these ruptures are not clinically significant and do not lead to hemodynamic instability. However, there is the potential for a life-threatening rupture, and the implanter should be prepared to handle this on an emergent basis by placing covered stents or referring for immediate surgery.

Stent fractures. Stent fracture of the valve frame is a recognized complication of Melody valve implantation and may lead to loss of structural integrity and recurrent obstruction requiring reintervention. Cabalka et al analyzed data from the prospective North American and European Melody valve trials and showed that prestenting decreased the risk of stent fracture and that this risk was further reduced by the placement of multiple prestents.[34] Therefore, it has become standard procedure when placing a Melody valve to prestent until there is no or minimal (<1 mm) recoil of the stent.

Coronary compression. This is a potential complication preventing percutaneous pulmonary valve implantation (PPVI) in approximately 5% of patients. This risk is present even for PPVI within bioprosthetic valves and therefore should always be assessed during the procedure. This is accomplished by simultaneously performing balloon angioplasty on the conduit (at the intended size of PPVI) while also assessing the coronary arteries with either ascending aortography or selective coronary angiography.

Endocarditis. Endocarditis has been reported for every type of bioprosthetic valve regardless of whether they are implanted surgically or percutaneously. This is a temporally related phenomenon, so the longer the patients with a PPVI are followed, the higher is the likelihood that an episode of endocarditis will be diagnosed.

Vascular complications. Reports of major vascular complications have been infrequent, with 8 events in 618 cases (1.1%; 95% CI, 0.5%-2.3%), but this may represent an issue for both smaller patients and those who undergo serial transcatheter interventions. Though typically femoral venous access has been used, the right internal jugular vein and subclavian vein have also been used even in relatively small patients.[32,33]

■ TROUBLESHOOTING

Management of Patients With Valvular Heart Disease After Valve Intervention and Suspected Complications

The clinical course of patients with prosthetic heart valves or repaired native valves will be determined by several factors, including ventricular function, atrial fibrillation (AF), pulmonary hypertension, and coronary artery disease, as well as by the development of valve-related complications. A valve intervention leaves the patient with either a prosthetic valve or a valve repair, often with an implanted device or other prosthetic material; hence, it does not eliminate valve disease. Patients with VHD will require serial evaluation after intervention for early postprocedural issues, long-term medical therapy, monitoring of the prosthetic valve or repair, and management of concurrent cardiac conditions and persistent symptoms or functional limitation. The interval between routine follow-up visits depends on the patient's valve type, the presence of residual heart disease, and other clinical factors.[35]

Persistent symptoms or the appearance of new symptoms occurs in many patients after valve intervention and is often a cause of hospitalization. The first step in evaluation is to assess valve function to ensure symptoms are not caused by persistent or recurrent stenosis, regurgitation,

or a valve complication. The most common complication early after surgical valve replacement is postoperative AF, which occurs in up to one-third of patients within 3 months of surgery. Other complications include stroke, vascular and bleeding complications, pericarditis, heart block requiring temporary or permanent pacing (especially after Aortic valve replacement [AVR]), HF, renal dysfunction, and infection. Complications after transcatheter interventions depend on the specific procedure but can include the need for permanent pacing, PVL, stroke, vascular complications, functional stenosis and residual valve dysfunction.[35]

Of the structural abnormalities, PPM, some types of dehiscence and PVL, infective endocarditis, and aortic dissection occur immediate in the postoperative period. The remaining complications occur remote from the postoperative period. Infective endocarditis and thrombus can occur anytime, but infective endocarditis is more common in the first 5 years and thrombus in the first year. Pannus is seen later, typically after 5 years. Late development of thrombus could be from underlying pannus. Structural failure and calcification are more common after 8 to 10 years.[36]

Risk factors associated with accelerated (<5 years) valve deterioration include young age (<60 years) at implantation, smoking, diabetes mellitus, chronic kidney disease, initial mean gradient ≥15 mmHg, and valve type.

Another step is to evaluate and treat any concurrent cardiac disease and noncardiac conditions that may be the cause of symptoms. Symptoms also may be attributable to irreversible consequences of valve disease, including LV systolic and diastolic dysfunction, pulmonary hypertension, and RV dysfunction; therefore, management of symptoms should be dependent of the underlying disease.[35]

When assessing a patient with suspected valvular dysfunction or postprocedure complication, it is important to obtain a detailed medical history including type and timing of intervention, baseline imaging studies including TTE, and medication history and adherence, especially to anticoagulation and antibiotics prophylaxis. Depending on the intervention that was done, potential complications (procedural or device related) may be consider and investigations should be done according to any suspicion.

Bioprosthetic or repaired native valve dysfunction will typically present with sudden onset of HF symptoms or a change in the auscultatory findings, and these symptoms may be more severe and abrupt in case of infective endocarditis or rupture of valve cups. There should be a high index of suspicion for mechanical valve dysfunction in the setting of CS, thromboembolic events, and/or hemolysis. Presentation may often be acute or subacute because of thrombus formation and more abrupt impairment of leaflet opening or closure. Repeat noninvasive assessment begins with TTE, comparison with the index postoperative study if available, and the use of other modalities as dictated by the clinical context and preliminary findings.[35]

Additional testing including laboratory values and other imaging modalities may be required on evaluation of suspected complications, and the early involvement of a multidisciplinary care team is highly recommended because some patients may require reintervention in the catheterization lab or the operating room.

Multimodality Imaging Use for Prosthetic Valves and Dysfunction

Transthoracic and Transesophageal Echocardiography

TTE after valve implantation or repair provides an assessment of the postprocedural results in a stable clinical state of the patient and can be used as a baseline comparison for any future changes. It provides hemodynamic measurements of transvalvular pressure gradients, velocities, and valve area, which can vary depending on different types of prosthetic heart valves and their size, which will aid in the detention of prosthetic dysfunction such as transvalvular and paravalvular leak, thrombosis or stenosis, and other potential complications. It also allows measurement of LV volume and LVEF, as well as evaluation of right heart structures. Occasionally, due to acoustic showing of a prosthetic valve, a TEE provides superior sensitivity for detection of prosthetic regurgitations, thrombus, pannus, abscess, or vegetation and is accurate for diagnosis of prosthetic mitral valve dysfunction. With mechanical valve obstruction, fluoroscopy or CT imaging can also be helpful for detection of reduced motion caused by pannus ingrowth or thrombus.[35]

Cine Fluoroscopy

Cine fluoroscopy is used as a problem-solving tool in prosthetic heart valve dysfunction and is particularly useful for evaluating morphology and mobility in patients with high echocardiography gradients. However, it does not allow the cause of prosthetic heart valve dysfunction to be established and does not provide hemodynamic or flow information, which limits its utility for assessing leaks.[36]

Computed Tomography

CT is performed after heart-rate control using β-blockers and uses a triphasic contrast material bolus technique. It is used to provide additional information on both mechanical and bioprosthetic valves, particularly for characterizing restricted leaflet, thrombus, pannus, vegetation, PVL, abscess, pseudoaneurysm, and fistulous connection. Prospective electrocardiographic (ECG) triggering is adequate for assessing morphology, but retrospective ECG gating is essential for dynamic 4-dimensional evaluation of the valve and functional quantification. A nonenhanced acquisition is useful for detecting calcifications and postsurgical changes, while a delayed phase (60-90 seconds) helps in evaluating abscess cavities with rim enhancement and thrombus. Coronary arteries and the relationship of cardiovascular structures to the sternum can also be evaluated. However, CT is not ideal if the patient has severe renal dysfunction, cardiac arrhythmia, or certain valve types (Björk-Shiley and Sorin monoleaflet).

Magnetic Resonance Imaging

MRI can be used for the same indications as CT when TTE is inadequate, when TEE is not possible or advisable, or typically when CT is contraindicated. MRI performs better with bioprosthetic than mechanical valves due to the artifacts with the latter. It is useful for assessment of complex hemodynamics and is particularly useful for prosthetic heart valves in the right heart.

Nuclear Medicine Techniques

Nuclear medicine techniques have a limited role in evaluating prosthetic heart valves, with limited data, and are mainly useful in evaluation of PHV infection and inflammation. Single-photon emission CT/CT with indium-111 oxime or technetium-99m HMPAO (hexamethylpropyleneamine oxime) and positron emission tomography (PET)/CT with fluorine-18 (^{18}F) fluorodeoxyglucose show increased activity with infection. While PET images can be acquired 1 hour after injection, SPECT requires early and late images. ^{18}F sodium fluoride PET/CT has shown promise in characterizing active tissue calcification and may play a future role in evaluation of bioprosthetic degeneration.[36]

REFERENCES

1. Zhang Y, Xiong T, Feng, Y. Current status and challenges of valvular heart disease interventional therapy. *Cardiol Discovery.* 2002;2(2):97-113.

2. Muller DWM, Farivar RS, Jansz P, et al. Transcatheter mitral valve replacement for patients with symptomatic mitral regurgitation. *J Am Coll Cardiol.* 2017;69(4):381-391.

3. Bora V, Brown KN, Lim MJ. *Catheter Management of Mitral Regurgitation*. [Updated 2022 Nov 27]. In: StatPearls [Internet]. Treasure Island, FL: StatPearls Publishing; 2022.

4. Akodad M, Schurtz G, Adda J, Leclercq F, Roubille F. Management of valvulopathies with acute severe heart failure and cardiogenic shock. *Arch Cardiovasc Dis.* 2019;112(12):773-780.

5. Ruiz CE, Kliger C, Perk G, et al. Transcatheter therapies for the treatment of valvular and paravalvular regurgitation in acquired and congenital valvular heart disease. *J Am Coll Cardiol.* 2015;66(2):169-183.

6. Schnitzler K, Hell M, Geyer M, Kreidel F, Münzel T, von Bardeleben RS. Complications following MitraClip implantation. *Curr Cardiol Rep.* 2021;23(9):131.

7. Gheorghe L, Ielasi A, Rensing BJWM, et al. Complications following percutaneous mitral valve repair. *Front Cardiovasc Med.* 2019;6:146.

8. Ghrair F, Omran J. Percutaneous mitral valve therapies: the old, current, and future. July 31, 2020. Accessed September 13, 2023. https://www.acc.org/latest-in-cardiology/articles/2020/07/31/08/28/percutaneous-mitral-valve-therapies

9. Rogers JH, Boyd WD, Smith TW, Bolling SF. Transcatheter mitral valve direct annuloplasty with the millipede IRIS ring. *Interv Cardiol Clin.* 2019;8(3):261-267.

10. Gheorghe L, Brouwer J, Wang DD, et al. Current devices in mitral valve replacement and their potential complications. *Front Cardiovasc Med.* 2020;7:531843.

11. Colli A, Adams D, Fiocco A, et al. Transapical NeoChord mitral valve repair. *Ann Cardiothorac Surg.* 2018;7(6):812-820.

12. Palacios IF. Percutaneous mitral balloon valvuloplasty: state of the art. *Mini-invasive Surg.* 2020;4:73.

13. Mahmaljy H, Tawney A, Young M. *Transcatheter Aortic Valve Replacement*. [Updated 2022 Nov 28]. In: StatPearls [Internet]. Treasure Island, FL: StatPearls Publishing; 2022. https://www.ncbi.nlm.nih.gov/books/NBK431075

14. Huang H, Kovach CP, Bell S, et al. Outcomes of emergency transcatheter aortic valve replacement. *J Interv Cardiol.* 2019;2019:7598581.

15. Fassa A, Himbert D, Vahanian A. Mechanisms and management of TAVR-related complications. *Nat Rev Cardiol.* 2013;10(12):685-695.

16. Chiarito M, Spirito A, Nicolas J, et al. Evolving devices and material in transcatheter aortic valve replacement: what to use and for whom. *J Clin Med.* 2022;11:4445.

17. Testa L, Rubbio AP, Casenghi M, et al. Transcatheter mitral valve replacement in the transcatheter aortic valve replacement era. *J Am Heart Assoc.* 2019;8(22):e013352.

18. Parikh PB, Kodali S. Transfemoral TAVR: balloon-expandable valves. In: Ailawadi G, Kron I, eds. *Catheter Based Valve and Aortic Surgery*. New York, NY: Springer; 2016. https://doi-org.eresources.mssm.edu/10.1007/978-1-4939-3432-4_2

19. Reul RM, Ramchandani MK, Reardon MJ. Transcatheter aortic valve-in-valve procedure in patients with bioprosthetic structural valve deterioration. *Methodist Debakey Cardiovasc J.* 2017;13(3):132-141.

20. Eugène M, Urena M, Abtan J, et al. Effectiveness of rescue percutaneous balloon aortic valvuloplasty in patients with severe aortic stenosis and acute heart failure. *Am J Cardiol.* 2018;121(6):746-750.

21. Williams T, Hildick-Smith DJR. Balloon aortic valvuloplasty: indications, patient eligibility, technique and contemporary outcomes. *Heart.* 2020;106:1102-1110.

22. Ng VG, Khalique OK, Nazif T, Patel A. Treatment of acute aortic insufficiency with a dedicated device. *JACC Case Rep.* 2021;3(4):645-649.

23. Bishop MA, Borsody K. *Percutaneous Tricuspid Valve Repair*. [Updated 2022 Oct 24]. In: StatPearls [Internet]. Treasure Island, FL: StatPearls Publishing; 2022. https://www.ncbi.nlm.nih.gov/books/NBK564430/

24. Zahr F, Chadderdon S, Song H, et al. Contemporary diagnosis and management of severe tricuspid regurgitation. *Catheter Cardiovasc Interv.* 2022;100:646-661.

25. Rogers JH, Bolling SF. The tricuspid valve: current perspective and evolving management of tricuspid regurgitation. *Circulation.* 2009;119(20):2718-2725.

26. Beckhoff F, Alushi B, Jung C, et al. Tricuspid regurgitation: medical management and evolving interventional concepts. *Front Cardiovasc Med.* 2018;5:49.

27. Kolte D, Elmariah S. Current state of transcatheter tricuspid valve repair. *Cardiovasc Diagn Ther.* 2020;10(1):89-97.

28. Matli K, Mahdi A, Zibara V, et al. Transcatheter tricuspid valve intervention techniques and procedural steps for the treatment of tricuspid regurgitation: a review of the literature. *Open Heart.* 2022;9:e002030.

29. Romeo JD, Bashline MJ, Fowler JA, et al. Current status of transcatheter tricuspid valve therapies. *Heart Int.* 2022;16(1):49-58.

30. Lauten A, Hans R. Figulla, Axel Unbehaun, Neil Fam, Joachim Schofer, Torsten Doenst, Joerg Hausleiter, Marcus Franz, Christian Jung, Henryk Dreger, David Leistner, Brunilda Alushi, Anja Stundl, Ulf Landmesser, Volkmar Falk, Karl Stangl and Michael Laule Originally published 14 Feb 2018 https://doi.org/10.1161/CIRCINTERVENTIONS.117.006061 Circulation: Cardiovascular Interventions. 2018;11:e006061

31. Goldberg YH, Ho E, Chau M, Latib A. Update on transcatheter tricuspid valve replacement therapies. *Front Cardiovasc Med.* 2021;8:619558.

32. O'Byrne ML, Gillespie MJ. Pulmonary insufficiency: melody valve. In: Ailawadi G, Kron I, eds. *Catheter Based Valve and Aortic Surgery.* New York, NY: Springer; 2016. https://doi-org.eresources.mssm.edu/10.1007/978-1-4939-3432-4_21

33. Balzer D. Pulmonary valve replacement for tetralogy of Fallot. *Methodist Debakey Cardiovasc J.* 2019;15(2):122-132.

34. Cabalka AK, Asnes JD, Balzer DT, et al. Transcatheter pulmonary valve replacement using the melody valve for treatment of dysfunctional surgical bioprostheses: A multicenter study. J Thorac Cardiovasc Surg. 2018 Apr;155(4):1712-1724.e1.

35. Otto CM, Nishimura RA, Bonow RO, et al. 2020 ACC/AHA guideline for the management of patients with valvular heart disease: a report of the American College of Cardiology/American Heart Association Joint Committee on Clinical Practice Guidelines. *Circulation.* 2021;143:e72-e227.

36. Rajiah P, Moore A, Saboo S, et al. Multimodality imaging of complications of cardiac valve surgeries. *RadioGraphics.* 2019;39(4):932-956.

CHAPTER 3

Coronary and Mechanical Circulatory Unit

• *Muhammad Khuram Nouman, MD; Muhammad Saad, MD;*
Tamir D. Vittorio; Gregory Serrao, MD; Fareeha Alavi

■ CASE PRESENTATION

A 62-year-old man came into the emergency department for sudden onset of angina that started 2 hours before the presentation and woke him up from sleep. He was known to have diabetes mellitus, hypertension, and hyperlipidemia. When the emergency medical service arrived, the electrocardiogram showed inferior wall ST-segment elevation myocardial infarction, and he was rushed to the hospital. En route, he continued to have chest pain that was not relieved by nitroglycerine; he was loaded with aspirin. His vital signs showed a blood pressure of 110/75 mmHg, a pulse of 75 bpm, and oxygen saturation of 98% on a 2-L nasal cannula, and the patient was afebrile. He was taken to the cardiac catheterization lab on hospital arrival for emergent revascularization. In the catheterization lab, he had a cardiac arrest with ventricular fibrillation. He was shocked and cardiopulmonary resuscitation (CPR) was initiated with no return of spontaneous circulation (ROSC). He was intubated and placed on mechanical ventilation. His initial blood gas showed pH of 7.01, PCO_2 of 65 mmHg, PaO_2 of 40% on fraction of inspired oxygen (FiO_2) 100%, and HCO_3 of 8. CPR was continued, and ROSC was achieved in 15 minutes with mean arterial pressure (MAP) around 55 mmHg and lactic acid of 12 mmole/liter with multiple pressers. A diagnostic coronary angiogram showed thrombotic occlusion of the right coronary artery (RCA). The decision was made to initiate venoarterial extracorporeal membrane oxygenation (VA-ECMO) given cardiogenic shock requiring percutaneous coronary intervention (PCI).

The patient was started on VA-ECMO via femoral cannulation with a flow rate of 3.5 to 4 L/min with intra-aortic balloon pump (IABP) insertion with 1:1 augmentation. He underwent PCI of the RCA with a drug-eluting stent placed and Thrombolysis in Myocardial Infarction (TIMI) III flow. His mixed venous oxygen saturation was maintained at 60% to 80%. The dobutamine and epinephrine drips were titrated to maintain a goal cardiac index greater than 2.2 L/min/m². Day 1 echocardiogram showed an ejection fraction of 20%, but patient hemodynamics continued to improve. Subsequently, he was able to be weaned off dobutamine and pressor. The repeat echocardiogram on day 6 showed an ejection fraction of 55% with central venous pressure (CVP) of 5 mmH_2O and pulmonary capillary wedge pressure (PCWP) of 12 mmH_2O. The patient was gradually weaned off extracorporeal membrane oxygenation (ECMO), and the patient was successfully extubated on the following day. He continued to feel better and was eventually discharged home.

■ HISTORICAL PERSPECTIVE

Before ECMO use in humans, the concept of a bypass machine was applied to cats by Gibbon in the late 1930s. He was able to support cats for up to 2 hours. However, further development could only be done after the start of the Second World War. Later in the 1950s, Gibbon successfully used the machine on dogs with an almost 90% survival rate. He was later able to successfully use the machine on an 18-year-old girl. However, his initial success was met with failures in later procedures, and he became pessimistic about the development and use of the heart-lung machine in humans. The story of the new ECMO circuit was led by 2 groups working concurrently, led by John Kirklin and Walton Lillehei.

In the 1960s, cardiopulmonary bypass was becoming more popular and considered a viable solution. However, the Gibbon heart-lung machine needed further modification. In 1967, the first heart transplant was performed; although it was unsuccessful, it was made possible by using cardiopulmonary bypass.

ECMO was used for the first time successfully in the early 1970s in a patient with severe lung injury after a motor vehicle accident, but the patient later died. In 1972, ECMO use in another patient finally led to the patient's survival. In 1974, ECMO was used in a newborn with meconium aspiration for 72 hours (about 3 days), and the baby survived to adulthood. After that, various studies showed poor survival outcomes with ECMO that led to further delays in the use and development of ECMO. The following decades were spent developing and modifying different ECMO parts. Between 1990 and 2000, polymethyl pentene oxygenators and centrifugal pumps were introduced. These developments led to fewer complications.

Extracorporeal Life Support Organization (ELSO) data supported using ECMO in newborns with heart and lung problems. The CESAR trial, which compared conventional ventilation with ECMO, further supported the use of ECMO. During the influenza pandemic in 2009, ECMO was used with over 70% survival rate in acute respiratory distress syndrome (ARDS) patients compared to conventional ventilation. In 2020, the utility of ECMO emerged during the COVID-19 pandemic.

■ MECHANISM OF ACTION

The basic principle of ECMO can be divided into 2 parts (Figure 3-3).

1. **Oxygenation.** This can be done by allowing gas exchange through an oxygenator.
2. **Pumping.** If the pumping component of the ECMO machine is used, it can aid cardiac pumping and replace cardiac function.

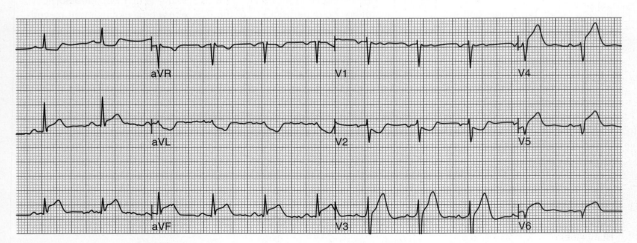

FIGURE 3-1. Electrocardiogram showing inferior wall ST-segment elevated myocardial infarction.

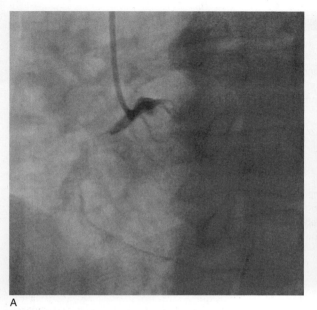
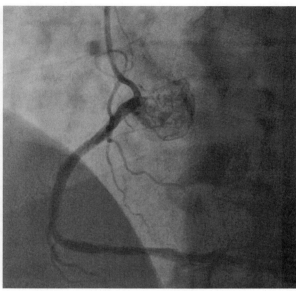

A

B

FIGURE 3-2. Coronary angiogram showing mid-RCA occlusion before and after PCI.

COMPONENTS OF ECMO

The important parts of an ECMO machine are listed in Table 3-2.

TYPES OF ECMO

ECMO can be divided into 2 major types (Figures 3-4 and 3-5).

1. **Venovenous ECMO (VV-ECMO).** Two cannulation approaches are used: (1) femoral vein and right internal jugular are used for infusion, and (2) both femoral veins are used for drainage and perfusion.

2. **Venoarterial ECMO (VA-ECMO).** Femoral vein (outflow) and femoral, axillary, and carotid arteries (inflow) are used for perfusion.

ECMO CIRCUIT

Once a patient qualifies for ECMO, the process starts with the percutaneous placement of a cannula, ideally in the operating room. The patient is started on intravenous heparin to avoid thrombus formation in the circuit. Once the target anticoagulation therapy of 300 to 350 seconds is achieved, the patient is initiated on ECMO.

The tubing of the ECMO is transparent to allow visual monitoring of the blood color and any clot formation in the circuit. In addition, tubing uses heparin-coated material to avoid any clot formation. There is also a bridging

■ TABLE 3-1. Hemodynamic Parameters		
Parameters	**Parameters on Day 1 on VA-ECMO**	**Parameters on Weaning**
Cardiac Index	1.6 L/min/m^2	2.8 L/min/m^2
CVP	14 mmHg	5 mmHg
PCWP	25 mmHg	9 mmHg
MAP	55 mmHg	85 mmHg
Lactic acid	12 mmol/L	1 mmol/L
Creatinine	1.3 mg/dL	0.9 mg/dL
Hemoglobin	12.2 g/dL	10.2 g/dl

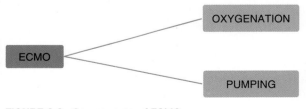

FIGURE 3-3. Components of ECMO.

■ **TABLE 3-2. Components of ECMO**

Part	Comments
Catheter 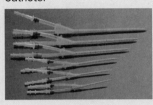	• Placed and removed under strict aseptic technique • Should be placed under ultrasound or fluoroscopic guidance • Ideally should be done in the operating room
Tubing 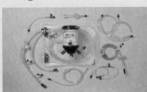	• Connects various components of ECMO • Usually heparin-coated to prevent clots • Act as a bridge between venous and arterial lines to allow blood recirculation • Side ports to allow blood sampling or Renal Replacement Therapy (RRT)
Pump 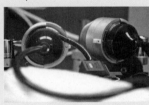	• Move the blood through the ECMO circuit • Vein → pump → oxygenator → vein (VV-ECMO) • Vein → pump → oxygenator → artery (VA-ECMO); this bypasses the heart • If no pump is used, then the artery-venous circuit is driven by the patient's blood pressure
Oxygenator 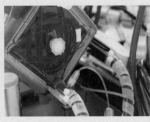	• Artificial lung • Has a membrane that allows gas exchange • Oxygen transfer is directly proportional to the surface area of the membrane, time of contact with blood, and oxygen delivered to the oxygenator
Heat exchanger 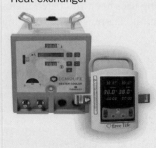	• Keeps the patient warm • Can adjust or cool body temperature in cardiac arrest patients • Uses water in the circuit to adjust temperatures

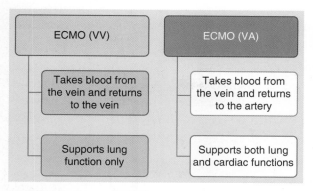

FIGURE 3-4. Types of ECMO.

pumps and centrifugal pumps. However, centrifugal pumps are more efficacious because of less hemolysis and anticoagulation requirements than roller pumps. A pump creates a negative pressure that allows the entrance of blood into the circuit from the patient. This blood then moves through the pump that makes positive pressure, allowing blood flow in the return circuit. The pump's function largely depends on preload and afterload in the ECMO circuit. Any occlusion in the circuit can affect the flow of blood.

Blood then enters the oxygenator, which is also called an artificial lung. The artificial lung is a membrane oxygenator that allows oxygen and carbon dioxide exchange. Gas enters the oxygenator via an oxygen blender with a flowmeter that regulates the gas flow. After oxygenation of the blood in the oxygenator, it is imperative to thermoregulate the blood to ensure that the patient is warm. Various mechanisms are available, but the commonly

in the tubing between arterial and venous lines that allows blood recirculation within the ECMO circuit.

A pump acts as a heart for blood circulation through the ECMO circuit. Common types of pumps are roller

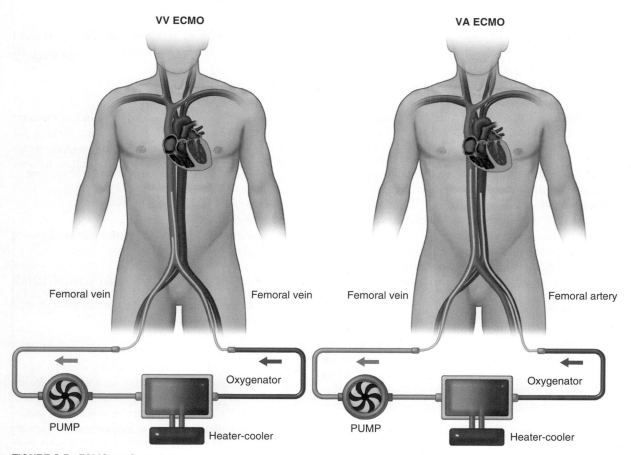

FIGURE 3-5. ECMO configuration.

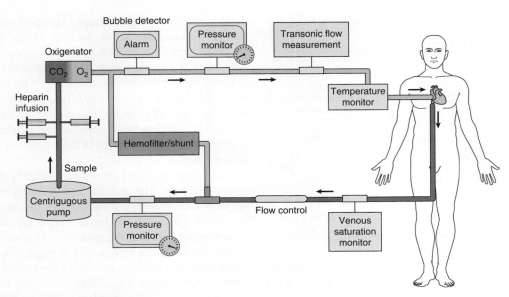

FIGURE 3-6. ECMO circuit diagram. (See color insert.)

used mechanism is circulating warm water around the oxygenator.

After rewarming the blood, the oxygenated blood returns to the patient via return cannulation.

■ CLINICAL CONSIDERATIONS AND DECISION MAKING

ECMO should be considered in young patients with acutely deteriorating clinical status with potentially reversible cardiac and respiratory failure despite maximal intensive treatment.

The patient should ideally be identified quickly before end-organ damage occurs.

Extracorporeal cardiopulmonary resuscitation (ECPR) can be considered in certain situations with cardiac arrest if the facility is equipped with the technology.

Outcome Prediction Scores

There are certain outcomes scores derived from the ELSO registry that can be used by physicians for decision making to predict survival when considering patents for ECMO initiation. These scores or calculators cannot be used to follow patients on ECMO. The following are a few risk prediction calculators that can be found online:

- SAVE score for VA-ECMO (https://www.elso.org/SaveScore/Index.html)

- RESP score for VV-ECMO (http://www.respscore.com)
- PIPER score (https://www.elso.org/ecmo-resources/piperscore.aspx)

ECMO Exit Strategy

Because ECMO is a temporary resuscitation measure for a failing heart or lung, the decision making for ECMO placement should include the overall prognosis of the patient along with the following exit strategies:

- Bridge to recovery
- Bridge to decision
- Bridge to durable support (left ventricular assist device or transplant)

■ INDICATIONS AND CONTRAINDICATIONS

Table 3-3 demonstrates important indications and contraindications of VA-/VV-ECMO.

Concept of ECPella and ECPR

In patients with ST-segment elevated myocardial infarction with cardiogenic shock, the management of left ventricular (LV) unloading can be done by placement of Impella with VA-ECMO. This can be done in the catheterization lab under fluoroscopic guidance after assessing LV distension and vascular anatomy.

■ TABLE 3-3. Indications and Contraindications of VA-/VV-ECMO

Indications	Contraindications
Cardiogenic shock	**Absolute contraindication for venoarterial ECMO**
• Acute myocardial infarction	• Irreversible cardiac dysfunction or other organ dysfunction such as liver cirrhosis or end-stage renal disease (with no arrangement for the transplant)
• Post–myocardial infarction complications, including ventricular wall rupture, refractory arrhythmias, and papillary muscle rupture	• Severe neurologic trauma or recent neurologic procedure
• Refractory to traditional therapy	• Inadequate vascular access
• Nonresponsive to IABP	• Aortic dissection
• Stress cardiomyopathy	• Unwitnessed cardiac arrest
Pulmonary	• Severe pulmonary hypertension and right ventricular failure
• Severe ARDS	• Immunosuppression
• Status asthmaticus	• Age >70-75
• Alveolar proteinosis	**Relative contraindication**
• Severe smoke inhalation injury	• Contraindications to anticoagulation
• Post–lung transplant failure	• Poor life expectancy
• Severe pulmonary embolism	• Disseminated malignancy
Infections	• Aggressive mechanical ventilation >7 days
• Myocarditis	• Severe metabolic acidosis
• Severe sepsis with cardiac depression	• Pulmonary fibrosis
Trauma	• Deranged coagulation profile
• Myocardial contusion	
• Major vessel trauma	
• Pulmonary contusion	
• Massive hemoptysis	
• Pulmonary hemorrhage	
Surgical	
• Bridge to heart or lung transplant	
• Posttransplant acute graft rejection	
• Postcardiotomy shock	
Pregnancy	
• Peripartum cardiomyopathy	

Another scenario is VA-ECMO placement in witnessed cardiac arrest patients with bedside ECMO cannulation and CPR. In this situation, Impella can be placed in the catheterization lab after LV end diastolic pressure assessment.

■ ROUTINE MONITORING AND FOLLOW-UP IN ECMO PATIENTS

The ECMO care team consists of a critical care physician, ECMO specialist nurses and respiratory therapists, perfusionist, cardiac surgeon, and pharmacists.

Best Practice Guidelines in ECMO Patients

- Daily echocardiogram
- Daily hemodynamics using pulmonary artery catheter
- Right radial arterial line
- Noninvasive cerebral oximeter
- Peripheral perfusion
- Therapeutic anticoagulation (using heparin with target partial thromboplastin time between 45 and 70 seconds)
- Labs every 4 to 6 hours (complete blood count, blood gas, electrolytes, lactate, creatinine)

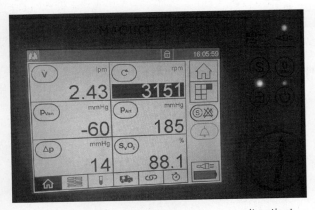

FIGURE 3-7. ECMO console in coronary care unit patient. (See color insert.)

- Transfuse if hemoglobin is less than 8 g/dL (in some centers <10 g/dL)
- Keep pH between 7.35 and 745 and platelets above 50,000

Daily Terms Used for ECMO Patients

Although every institute has their own standard protocols for initiation and monitoring of ECMO patients, Figure 3-8 shows the terms used universally for ECMO patients.

Oxygenation Issues in ECMO

VV-ECMO

- Blood and oxygen to the membrane oxygenator determine partial pressure of oxygen (PO_2),

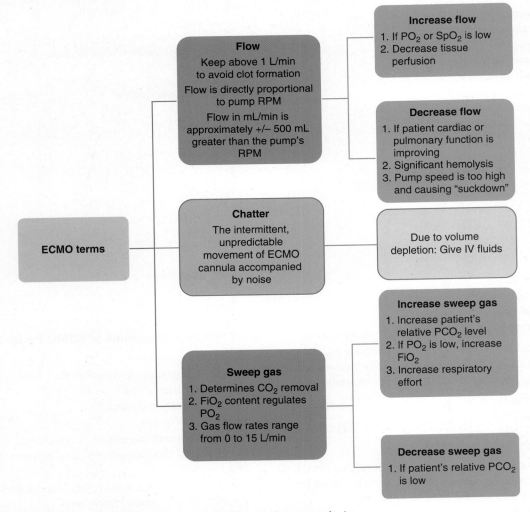

FIGURE 3-8. Daily terms used in ECMO patients. RPM, revolutions per minute.

1. Insufficient oxygenator flow
2. Membrane issue

- The cause of a low PO_2 must be determined, but oxygen delivery can be improved by:
  1. Increasing sweep gas FiO_2
  2. Increasing the ventilator's FiO_2 setting

VA-ECMO

- VA-ECMO mixes blood from the oxygenator and the patient's heart and lungs.
- The patient's right radial artery measures PO_2.
- If the patient has poor pulmonary function, the oxygenator's well-oxygenated blood will mix with the native pulmonary circulation's poorly oxygenated blood, causing hypoxemia.
- Increasing flow reduces the patient's pulmonary vasculature blood flow, correcting low PO_2.
- Increasing sweep gas FiO_2 can correct low PO_2, but the source must be investigated (see troubleshooting section for more details).

Membrane Gases

- Compare pre- and postmembrane gases to evaluate the membrane oxygenator.
- The perfusionist draws 40 to 70 mmHg premembrane gas from a port before the blood reaches the oxygenator.
- The perfusionist draws 300 to 500 PO_2 postmembrane gas from a port after the blood leaves the oxygenator.
- Postmembrane gas PO_2 should be substantially greater than that of premembrane gas.
- A low PO_2 rise indicates a membrane issue.
- In VV-ECMO, if the premembrane PO_2 is significantly higher than expected, the drainage cannula is "recirculating" oxygenated blood from the return cannula instead of allowing it to perfuse the patient's organs (see troubleshooting section for more details).

Monitoring of ECMO

Because the ECMO circuit removes blood from the body and returns the blood after going through specific processes back to the body, many complications can happen in the ECMO circuit. This requires continuous monitoring by a team that is well trained in the handling of ECMO. Trained staff can detect tubing or clot formation kinks by visual inspection. The ECMO circuit and patient must be monitored simultaneously for earlier detection of problems.

Any occlusion or thrombus formation in the circuit can be detected by doing 2 things.

1. Visual inspection of the tubing
2. Pressure monitoring

Pressure monitoring can be done at 3 different locations in the ECMO circuit:

1. Before the blood enters the pump
2. After the blood leaves the pump and before it enters the oxygenator
3. After the blood leaves the oxygenator

An increase in pressure indicates either occlusion or thrombus formation.

Monitoring of Oxygenator

Blood gas monitoring can detect a failing oxygenator.

Monitoring Blood Flow Rate Through the Tubing

This can be monitored using an ultrasonic flow meter; any decrease in the blood flow leads to blood accumulation and clot formation.

■ TROUBLESHOOTING

Table 3-4 summarizes how to troubleshoot ECMO alarms and flow-related issues.

■ WEANING FROM ECMO

Table 3-5 provides steps for weaning from ECMO.

■ COMPLICATIONS

Table 3-6 shows a list of complications related to ECMO.

■ FUTURE OF ECMO

- The current cannulation system will be modified to allow more patient mobility.
- Current ECMO circuits have an artificial lung that is square in shape; future ECMO circuits will contain round-shaped artificial lungs to reduce blood stagnation and thrombus formation.
- The use of nitric oxide or platelet inhibitors will become more common to prevent platelet adhesions or aggregation.

■ **TABLE 3-4. ECMO Troubleshooting**

Problem	Alarms/Indicators	Solution
Kinking of cannula	Low flow alarm	Reposition patient, change cannula site
Cannula site blood loss	Low flow alarm	Manual pressure, local epinephrine injection
Circuit thrombosis	Low flow alarm	Adequate anticoagulation
Circuit rupture	Hypoxemia	Clamp the circuit, CPR, replace the circuit
Pump failure	Low flow alarm/hypoxemia	Check alarms, adjust pump's RPM, replacement
Air embolism	Low flow alarm/hypoxemia	Clamp the circuit, start CPR, and remove air from the circuit
LV distension (VA-ECMO, poor LV reserve, and increased afterload increase blood pooling and backflow in LV, leading to pulmonary edema)	CXR with pulmonary edema An echo with worsening LV function and minimal aortic opening Elevated PCWP and low cardiac output	Improve forward flow Increase pressers and inotropes Increase diuresis IABP or Impella/ECPella placement Surgical approaches include atrial septostomy
Dropping flows	Low flow alarm	Make sure the pump speed is at the target RPM Check for kink and clot and repeat CXR or echo for the position Surgical consultation
Chatter (in VA-ECMO, rattling movement of venous drainage cannula)	Noise	Lower RPM temporarily Improve hydration and restore the pump speed to reassess Repeat CXR and echo and assess for increased intrathoracic or intra-abdominal pressure Kink or malposition
Recirculation (in 2-site VV-ECMO, oxygenated blood is sucked in by venous cannula, causing persistent hypoxemia)	Low SaO_2 and high SpO_2 (preoxygenator saturation)	Increase the distance between the drainage and reinfusion ports, with a target separation distance of approximately 15 cm Add a drainage cannula Switch to dual lumen or bicaval cannula
The harlequin syndrome, north-south syndrome (differential cyanosis occurs in peripheral VA-ECMO due to retrograde flow leading to the watershed area where 2 flows meet, depending on LV function)	A right radial arterial line can help distinguish the watershed area; if pulse pressure in A-line is narrow, the watershed area is in the aortic root; if wide, it is after the innominate artery	Increase ECMO flow Improve native lung oxygenation Conversion of ECMO configuration to VV-A by adding a Y-connector to split arterial outflow to improve oxygenation in the pulmonary circulation
Limb ischemia	Assess cannulated leg periodically Biomarkers such as lactic acid and creatine kinase levels Trending tissue oxygen saturations using lower-extremity NIRS on the calf muscles	Placement of 6-F sheath distal to the arterial cannula in the common femoral artery or superficial femoral artery to provide antegrade femoral blood flow to the cannulated leg

Abbreviations: NIRS, near-infrared spectroscopy; RPM, revolutions per minute.

■ **TABLE 3-5. ECMO Weaning**

Weaning From VV-ECMO	Weaning From VA-ECMO
• Cause of cardiogenic shock resolved • 24-48 hours minimum on ECMO before weaning • MAP >70 mmHg • Decreased pressor requirement • Improved hemodynamic parameters, ie, CVP, MVO$_2$, PCWP, and LV ejection fraction, pulse pressure >30 mmHg, LVOT VTI >12 • Lactic acid level <2 mmole/liter	• Native lungs provide ≥70%-80% of oxygenation • Pulmonary compliance and airway resistance improved • FiO$_2$ on mechanical ventilator <60% • PCO$_2$ improved to adequate levels • Once the patient is ready, the sweep gas flow to the oxygenator is reduced to zero
• The flow is decreased stepwise down to around 1.0 L/min • Patient hemodynamics, pressure requirements, and clinical data are closely monitored • Cannulas are clamped and can be left in for up to 24 hours; heparin continued; if the patient tolerates it, then ECMO can be decannulated • Heparin can be discontinued 30-60 minutes before decannulation; judicious local anesthesia should be used	• Ventilator parameters monitored, including tidal volume, minute ventilation, and respiratory rate • Clinical signs of respiratory distress are closely monitored; serial blood gases were obtained • Flow does not need to be changed • Once off sweep, ECMO can be decannulated • Surgical purse-string sutures can be placed for hemostasis

Abbreviations: LVOT, left ventricular outflow tract; MVO$_2$, myocardial volume oxygen; VTI, velocity time integral.

■ **TABLE 3-6. ECMO Complications**

Device-Related Complications	Medical Complications	
Catheter Fistula formation Hemorrhage, eg, retroperitoneal, pericardial Air embolism Cardiac arrhythmias Dissection Decannulation Compartment syndrome	**Neurologic** Stroke Brain bleeding Brain death Seizures Sinus thrombosis	**Renal** Renal failure Electrolyte imbalance Capillary leak syndrome Fluid retention
Circuit-related complications Air embolism Thrombosis Infection Blood loss Hemolysis Pump failure Oxygenator failure Failure to regulate temperature Circuit obstruction	**Cardiac** Cardiac arrhythmias Ischemia Hypoperfusion-reperfusion injury Cardiac stunning **Pulmonary** Pulmonary hemorrhage Pneumothorax Pulmonary embolism Pneumonitis Pulmonary hypertension	**Infectious** Catheter site infection Bloodstream infection **Hematologic** Hemolysis Heparin-induced thrombocytopenia Disseminated intravascular coagulation Bleeding Thrombosis

SUGGESTED READINGS

Bartlett RH. ECMO: the next ten years. *Egypt J Crit Care Med.* 2016;4(1):7-10.

Figueroa Villalba CA, McMullan DM, Reed RC, Chandler WL. Thrombosis in extracorporeal membrane oxygenation (ECMO) circuits. *ASAIO J.* 2022;68(8):1083-1092.

Sidebotham D. Troubleshooting adult ECMO. *J Extra Corpor Technol.* 2011;43(1):27-32.

Vuylsteke A, Brodie D, Combes A, Fowles J, Peek G. The ECMO circuit. In:*ECMO in the Adult Patient (Core Critical Care).* Cambridge University Press; 2017:25-57.

Abbreviations

ARDS: Acute respiratory distress syndrome
CPR: Cardiopulmonary resuscitation
CVP: Central venous pressure
CXR: Chest x-ray
ECPR: Extracorporeal cardiopulmonary resuscitation
ECMO: Extracorporeal membrane oxygenation
FiO_2: Fraction of inspired oxygen
IABP: Intra-aortic balloon pump
LV: Left ventricular
MAP: Mean arterial pressure
PaO_2: Arterial oxygen pressure
PCI: Percutaneous coronary intervention
PCWP: Pulmonary capillary wedge pressure
PO_2: Partial pressure of oxygen
RCA: Right coronary artery
ROSC: Return of spontaneous circulation
VA-ECMO: Venoarterial extracorporeal membrane oxygenation
VV-ECMO: Venovenous extracorporeal membrane oxygenation

CHAPTER 4

Cardiogenic Shock: Temporary Mechanical Circulatory Support Devices

• *Angel de la Cruz, MD; Sai Vishnuvardhan Allu, MD; Muhammad Saad, MD; Umesh Gidwani, MD*

■ CASE PRESENTATION

A 56-year-old woman with hypertension and hyperlipidemia presented to the emergency room complaining of sudden-onset central chest pain and shortness of breath. She was found to have an inferior ST-segment elevation myocardial infraction. She was immediately taken to the cardiac catheterization laboratory and received a drug-eluting stent in the right coronary artery with Thrombolysis in Myocardial Infarction (TIMI) grade III flow. Her heart rate was 115 bpm, and blood pressure was 80/60 mmHg. Dopamine was initiated in the catheterization lab and was titrated to maximum dose. Her blood pressure did not improve, and she continued to feel short of breath. At this point, a Swan-Ganz catheter was placed, and her pulmonary capillary wedge pressure was 20 mmH$_2$O, right atrial pressure was 12 mmHg, and cardiac index was 1.9. Echocardiogram showed left ventricular ejection fraction of 45%, moderate to severe mitral regurgitation, and no pericardial effusion. She was initiated on intra-aortic balloon pump (IABP) and taken to the critical care unit. Her hemodynamics were stabilized initially, and she continued to improve on subsequent days. Her vasopressor requirements were decreased, and she was weaned off IABP.

■ KEY POINTS

- Temporary mechanical circulatory support can be used in cardiogenic shock patients to stabilize hemodynamics.
- Percutaneous right and left support devices are considered as a temporary measure to unload ventricles during the periprocedural period in high-risk cases.
- Efforts are ongoing to improve the pump flow, catheter caliber, and ease of placement.

■ TEMPORARY MECHANICAL CIRCULATORY DEVICES

Over the past decade, mechanical circulatory support (MCS) has emerged as an important focus in the management of cardiogenic shock. Multiple randomized and observational trials have been ongoing to study the impact of MCS on survival outcomes in shock patients. Although initially introduced as an emergency device, MCS now has a role in elective high-risk cases, perioperative management, and transplant cases. Depending on

TABLE 4-1. Types of Percutaneous MCS	
Left Ventricle Support Devices	**Right Ventricle Support Devices**
Pulsatile flow Intra-aortic balloon pump **Continuous flow** Micro-axial: Impella device Centrifugal: Tandem Heart Device, extracorporeal membrane oxygenation, percutaneous heart pump	**Continuous flow** Micro-axial: RV Impella (Impella RP system) Centrifugal: ProtekDuo System Percutaneous RV assist device: CentriMag Acute Circulatory Support System

the patient's clinical scenario and need for hemodynamic support and the operator's experience, several types of MCS are available (Table 4-1).

PERCUTANEOUS LEFT VENTRICLE CIRCULATORY SUPPORT DEVICES

Intra-Aortic Balloon Pump

There are several modalities to support pump failure in cardiogenic shock. Intra-aortic balloon pump (IABP) is one of the first MCS devices used in cardiac patients. IABP is a pulsatile intravascular left ventricular circulatory support system designed to provide cardiac output. It can be emergently placed percutaneously either at bedside or in the cardiac catheterization laboratory.

Historical Perspective

The concept of IABP was used in 1960 with external counterpulsation, which was later reintroduced as an internal device by Dr. Adrian Kantrowitz. Its use became more popular after observational and registry data showed its effective role in coronary perfusion and improvement in cardiac output. However, the IABP-SHOCK II trial did not show any mortality benefit in shock patients. Based on these data, IABP placement has been downgraded from class I to class IIb in US and European guidelines. Currently, there is a limited role for IABP in shock, transplant, and angina management.

Mechanism of Action

The IABP is synchronized with the cardiac cycle and arterial waveform to provide synchronized counterpulsation and to improve myocardial function by increasing myocardial oxygen supply and decreasing myocardial oxygen demand. Main triggers for its function are the electrocardiogram (ECG) and pressure waves. The balloon inflates in diastole, hence helping in coronary filling, and deflates during systole, allowing peripheral perfusion. It provides a support of 0.5 L/min.

Because inflation and deflation of the IABP coincide with the closing and opening of the aortic valve, the IABP will be triggered to deflate during systole, when the peak of the R wave is sensed. Subsequently, IABP inflation will be triggered to occur in the middle of the T wave. During cases of poor electrocardiographic quality or arrhythmias, the ECG triggering mode becomes less reliable.

The pressure trigger mode is also often used. During this mode, the arterial pressure waveform is used to trigger IABP inflation and deflation. On the pressure waveform, the closure of the aortic valve corresponds with the dicrotic notch while the opening corresponds to the point immediately before the systolic upstroke. The IABP augmentation coincides with the opening and closing of the aortic valve. Other possible triggers include an "operator mode," which is an internal trigger, as well as pacer triggers.

The device can be placed on different frequencies. If placed on 1:1 mode, the device will support every single heartbeat. If placed on 1:2, the device will support every other heartbeat (Figure 4-1). And, if placed on 1:3, the device will support every third heartbeat. The IABP augments coronary perfusion pressure by increasing aortic

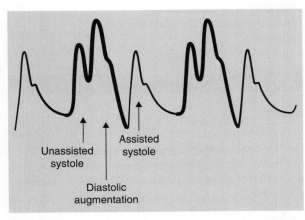

FIGURE 4-1. IABP with 1:2 augmentations. IABP inflation happens immediately after the aortic valve closes. IABP deflation occurs immediately before the aortic valve opens.

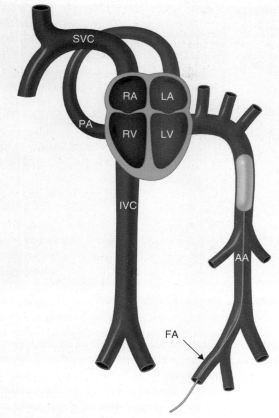

FIGURE 4-2. Configuration of IABP. AA, ascending artery; FA, femoral artery; IVC, inferior vena cava; LA, left atrium; LV, left ventricle; PA, pulmonary artery; RA, right atrium; RV, right ventricle; SVC, superior vena cava.

■ **TABLE 4-2. Contraindications for the Use of IABP**	
Absolute Contraindications	**Relative Contraindications**
Aortic regurgitation	Septic shock
Aortic dissection	Abdominal aortic
Aortic stent	aneurysm
Chronic end-stage	Peripheral vascular
heart disease with no	disease
expected recovery	Tachyarrhythmia

in urgent procedures. The contraindications are summarized in Table 4-2.

Technique

- After implementation of standard sterile techniques, a drape is placed.
- Access site can be either the femoral artery or axillary artery.
- Ultrasound-guided or fluoroscopic access is obtained using the Seldinger technique, and an 8-F sheath is placed.
- IABP is inserted and mounted using a premeasured length on a safe spot in the aorta by using fluoroscopy, transesophageal echocardiography, or X-ray.
- IABP is initiated in diastole timed with ECG or arterial waveform.

Equipment

IABP consists of 2 components:

1. Arterial cannulation catheter mounted with the helium inflation balloon. The balloon is made of polyurethane membrane with vascular catheter.
2. Console machine with gas pump to inflate pump.

Weaning IABP

- Once the hemodynamics and clinical parameters are improved, IABP can be switched to 2:1 or 3:1 configuration and the clinical situation should be reassessed.
- Continue anticoagulation, and once planning to remove IABP, heparin can be held for 30 minutes.
- Before pulling out, stop the IABP so the balloon is deflated and then pullout the IABP from the sheath.
- Remove the sheath and hold pressure on the femoral artery for hemostasis.

diastolic pressure and decreasing the left ventricular end-diastolic pressure. The decrease in oxygen demand is explained by a decrease in afterload due to the active balloon deflation at the beginning of systole, increasing forward blood flow through a vacuum effect (See Figure 4-2).

Indications and Contraindications

As discussed, IABP is one of the most widely used cardiac support devices. It assists in providing temporary coronary and systemic perfusion. This device is indicated in cases of acute myocardial infarction, cardiogenic shock, acute mitral regurgitation, and ventricular septal defect, as well as in cases of preoperative stabilization for coronary artery bypass grafting. It may also be used as a bridge to transplantation, for hemodynamic instability during percutaneous coronary intervention (PCI), and sometimes in cases of poor ejection fraction

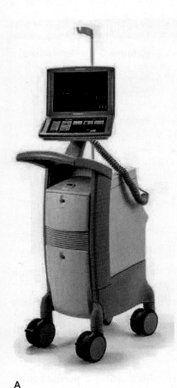

A

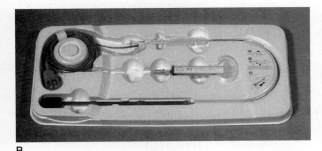

B

FIGURE 4-3. A, B. Equipment of IABP.

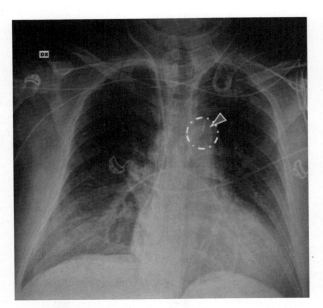

FIGURE 4-4. Chest X-ray showing IABP.

Complications

There are many complications associated with IABP insertion. Based on multiple studies, the most common complications are vascular injury, infection, and balloon malfunction. Vascular complications include ischemia to the visceral organs, extremities, and spinal cord and cerebrovascular accidents. There is also the possibility of arterial laceration, aneurysm and pseudoaneurysm, arterial dissection, and hemorrhage and hematoma. Other possible complications are those related to the balloon itself or its rupture. Gas embolism, hemolysis, and thrombocytopenia may occur.

Patients should be closely monitored for signs of limb ischemia. Close monitoring of clinical status and vital signs is key to appropriately identify complications and address them in a timely manner. In general, the main risk factors for developing complications related to the IABP insertion are peripheral vascular disease, diabetes mellitus, and age more than 70 years. Other possible risk factors are female gender, smoking, and obesity. Patients with low cardiac output state or cardiogenic shock are also at elevated risk.

Troubleshooting

In general, it is important to make sure the device is properly connected to a power source and that the tubing is intact. Relieving kinks, if any, is also important, as well as checking IABP markings and ensuring all the alarms are on.

There are a number of issues that may arise with IABP. One of the most common issues is the inability to sense trigger mode. The management for this is to switch to an alternative mode of triggering and/or to reconnect the ECG leads or pressure cable. Another issue that may arise is a low helium level on the machine, which is

■ TABLE 4-3. Complications of IABP		
Procedural Complications	Technical Complications	Hemodynamic Complications
Vascular insult/ hematoma/ thrombosis	Balloon rupture	Tachycardia
Kink in tubing	Balloon malposition	Aortic regurgitation
Limb ischemia	Loss of power supply	Aortic dissection

managed by replacing the cylinder. If there is a failure within the IABP console/computer, an electrical malfunction or blood in the condensers needs to be ruled out.

Another problem commonly described is when the augmentation is below the limit set, which may activate the alarm sign. If that is the case, clinical status needs to be addressed, and it may be necessary to lower the alarm limit. However, if there is a change in clinical status or hemodynamics, proceed to treat the clinical condition accordingly and search for signs of balloon displacement.

Future Directions
Although the use of IABP has recently been limited, efforts have been ongoing to improvise it for long-term ambulatory placement, especially in advance heart failure patients awaiting destination therapy.

Impella System

Impella system is an intravascular microaxial pump designed to deliver cardiac output from the left ventricle to the aorta. It can be placed by either percutaneous or surgical approach depending on the clinical situation.

Historical Perspective
The concept of the Impella device was initially introduced in 1985 by American physician Dr. Richard Wampler as the Hemopump. The device was first implanted in 1988; however, it did not receive commercial value due to the lack of improvement in outcomes. In 1991, the same concept was modified by German scientists Siess and colleagues who modified the pump and impeller. Based on these changes, the device was used

in acute myocardial infarction patients and showed improvement in infarct size. This observation led to the approval of the Impella system in Europe and the United States. Based on several small observational trials and registry data, Impella placement in cardiogenic shock patients may help improve mortality, but this has not yet been proven by any randomized controlled trial. The role of Impella 2.5 in high-risk PCI was shown in the PROTECT-II trial with no mortality benefit after 30 days; however, a trend toward improved outcomes was observed after 90 days.

Mechanism of Action
In general, the main idea of Impella is to reduce the ventricular work and provide the circulatory support necessary to allow cardiac recovery and early assessment of residual myocardial function. The hemodynamic support provided by Impella is due to a flow and pressure augmentation that leads to improved cardiac power output. The forward flow achieved clinically is dependent on the pump support level setting (P) and the pressure gradient between the aorta and the left ventricle. P setting ranges from P1 to P7. Higher P levels or lower pressure gradients will result in higher flow augmentation.

By decreasing the end-diastolic volume and end-diastolic pressure, Impella decreases the mechanical work and the wall tension of the left ventricle, which, in turn, decreases the oxygen demand. At the same time, by increasing the blood flow and the aortic pressure, there is an increase in oxygen supply and cardiac power output.

The net effect of the Impella is to unload the demand of myocardial oxygen and to augment the supply of oxygen through an increase in coronary blood flow. There have been many studies that have generally reported a 60% to 70% improvement in the net change of oxygen demand-supply ratio, compared with a 10% to 20% improvement with IABP alone.

Indications and Contraindications
Impella has a catheter that sits on the left ventricle, with an inlet that should be 3.5 to 5.5 cm from the aortic valve. There are many different types of Impella devices, including Impella 2.5; Impella CP, which provides a flow support of around 3.5 L/min; Impella 5.0, which provides a support of 5 L/min; and Impella 5.5, which provides a support of 5.5 to 6.0 L/min.

■ TABLE 4-4. Types of Impella

Impella Type	Sheath Size	Access	Flow (L/min)
Impella 2.5	13 F	Percutaneous femoral/axillary artery	2.5
Impella CP	14 F	Percutaneous femoral/axillary artery	3.5
Impella 5.0	23 F	Femoral/axillary artery surgical cutdown	5
Impella LP	Not applicable	Inserted directly in ascending aorta	5.3
Impella 5.5	23 F	Femoral/axillary artery surgical cutdown	5.5

The Impella 2.5 and Impella CP are temporary ventricular support devices that are indicated for use during high-risk PCIs in hemodynamically stable patients with severe coronary artery disease (CAD) to prevent hemodynamic instability due to repetitive episodes of reversible myocardial ischemia.

The Impella 2.5, Impella CP, and Impella 5.0 are ventricular support devices that are intended for short-term use (usually a maximum of 4-6 days) and are indicated in the treatment of ongoing cardiogenic shock that occurs immediately following acute myocardial infarction or open-heart surgery or in the setting of cardiomyopathy, such as myocarditis.

The main contraindications for Impella placement are mural thrombus in the left ventricle, moderate to severe aortic insufficiency, significant aortic valve stenosis, mechanical aortic valve, cardiac tamponade, presence of ventricular or atrial septal defect, and severe peripheral arterial disease that precludes the placement of the Impella catheter.

Equipment
There are 2 components of the Impella device:

1. Cannula/catheter that consists of 6-F pigtail attached at the distal end of the inlet cannula. The inlet area withdraws blood and shifts it to the motor system at the distal end near the outlet area. The outlet area is located on the ascending aorta, through which blood exits to the body.
2. Automated Impella controller consists of an interface to guide catheter management, serves as backup power supply, and purges the catheter. (See Figure 4-5.)

Technique
- After sterile femoral artery access, a pigtail diagnostic catheter is inserted in a retrograde fashion over a 0.035 stiff guidewire through the aorta and aortic valve and positioned in the left ventricle.

- Remove the guidewire and insert 0.018 guidewire, over which the pigtail catheter is removed and the Impella catheter is inserted under fluoroscopic guidance.
- Position the inlet area 3.5 cm below the aortic valve and in the mid-ventricle guided by fluoroscopy. Initiate the flow by following prompts on the automated controller.
- Once position is confirmed, the Impella can be secured by surgical sutures.
- Vascular anatomy using an angiogram should be assessed and needs to be part of the discussion before Impella placement.
- After insertion of the catheter, heparin should be initiated with a target partial thromboplastin time between 50 and 70 seconds.
- Before transferring the patient to the intensive care unit, remove the peel-away sheath and replace with repositioning sheath.
- The axillary approach can be used for patients requiring long-term support and help in mobility.
- Impella 5, 5.5, and LP can be surgically or transcavally placed using a cutdown and a vascular graft.

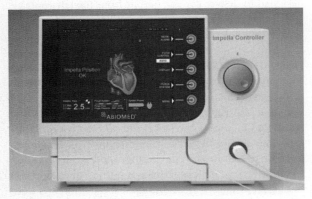

FIGURE 4-5. Impella controller. (See color insert.)

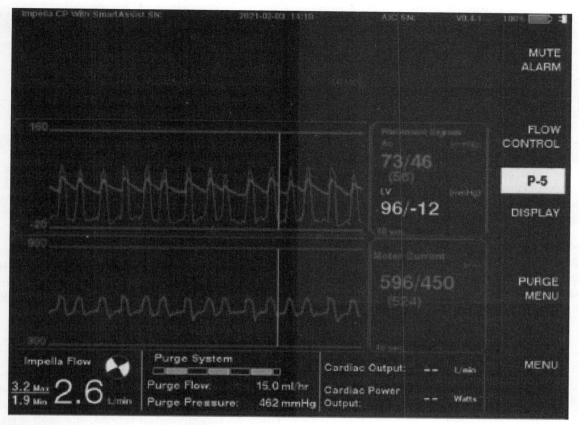

FIGURE 4-6. Placement screen. (See color insert.)

Weaning from Impella (Figure 4-7)

Impella weaning can be initiated once hemodynamic parameters are improving (including cardiac power output, urine output, lactic acid, and pressor/inotropic requirement). Reduce Impella P level every hour and continue to check hemodynamic parameters. Keep the lowest P level at P2 before explant. If hemodynamic parameters deteriorate at any level, uptitrate the inotrope for early weaning and then increase P level.

Complications

The possible complications related to the use of Impella are similar to those related to IABP. In a similar fashion, vascular complications are common. Limb ischemia is reported to occur in 0.07% to 10% of patients based on different studies. It is important to keep in mind that after Impella placement patients require continuous monitoring to manage these complications, if they occur.

Vascular injury requiring surgery is reported to occur in 1.3% to 2% of cases. Access site bleeding occurs relatively often, which is reported to occur in 2% to 40% of cases, as well as hemolysis, which is reported to occur in 10% to 46% of cases. As a result, hemolysis labs plasma-free hemoglobin, lactate dehydrogenase, haptoglobin, and bilirubin) should be checked frequently.

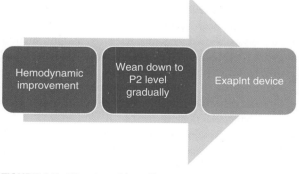

FIGURE 4-7. Weaning of Impella.

Other complications that are less common include major bleeding (0.05%-50%), hemorrhagic and ischemic cerebrovascular accidents (2%-6%), sepsis (0.16%-19%), device migration (0.05%-23%), and device malfunction (0.16%-17%). Regarding the last 2 complications mentioned, it is important to keep in mind that they could lead to injury to the aortic valve and mitral regurgitation secondary to injury to the papillary muscles. In patients with ischemic cerebrovascular accident, there may be associated risk of hemorrhagic transformation due to the anticoagulation.

In addition, because the catheter sits in the left ventricle, there is a theoretical risk of development of cardiac arrhythmias, for which the patients need to be closely monitored as well.

Troubleshooting

- If bleeding from the Impella is noted, confirm that the stopcock on the peel-away introducer or repositioning sheath is always kept in the closed position.
- It is also important to keep in mind that patients with Impella cannot undergo magnetic resonance imaging. If the lithium battery alarm turns on, management is replacement of the lithium battery.
- If there is air in purge system, initiate the De-Air Tool and follow instructions to remove the air from the system. If the battery is very low (power capacity of <15%), plug control into power.
- If an alarm is showing that the battery temperature is high (>60°C), switch to backup controller. Operating the Automated Impella Controller sometimes causes interference with ECG signals. Always make sure to check the electrode pads and leads for good fixation and contact. If the interference persists, consider activating the 50/100 Hz band-elimination filter or the 60/120 Hz band-elimination filter on the ECG device.
- Generally, for any suction alarm, malposition should be considered, and properly assess for cannula position by using echocardiography (Figure 4-8).
- Hemolysis should be considered as part of suction alarm troubleshooting and can be improved by hydration or device positioning.
- Right ventricle (RV) failure is another reason for continuous suction alarm and needs to be delineated as it may change the management.
- In general, it is important to make sure the device is properly connected to a power source and that the outside parts of the device are intact.

- It is also important to check the screen to ensure all the alarms are on and to access the alarm history screen for the menu to address any issues that have been reported.

Future Directions

- The Impella 9F system (Impella ECP) was approved by the US Food and Drug Administration (FDA) in August 2021. Inside the body, it can expand and may provide flow up to 5 L/min.
- Enrollment for the PROTECT-IV trial is ongoing to assess the role of Impella in assisted complex PCI to improve outcomes in high-risk patients with CAD and severely reduced left ventricular function.

Tandem Heart

Tandem Heart is a percutaneous extracorporeal centrifugal pump that can provide continuous flow for biventricular failure. It can be placed in the cardiac catheterization laboratory to support the failing heart.

Historical Perspective

The device was approved by the FDA in 2003 and, since then, it has been used to provide left ventricular support with flow as high as 4 L/min. Francesca et al described the first implantation of Tandem Heart as a short-term bridge for heart transplant in 2006. In a small study of 80 patients, Kar et al described that Tandem Heart use has a beneficial role in improving hemodynamic parameters in cardiogenic shock patients; however, considerable data

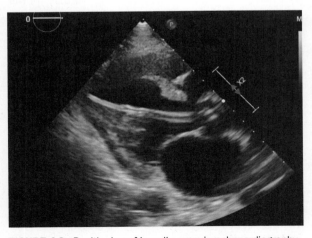

FIGURE 4-8. Positioning of Impella seen in echocardiography.

have shown higher adverse events such as bleeding. This limits the use of Tandem Heart because it requires greater expertise and monitoring.

Mechanism of Action

Tandem Heart works by simultaneously contributing blood flow to the aorta, working in conjunction with the left ventricle. Oxygenated blood is withdrawn from the left atrium, which is accessed by an inflow cannula inserted percutaneously through the femoral vein, up the inferior vena cava (IVC), into the right atrium, and then via transseptal puncture into the left atrium. Afterward, blood is pumped by a centrifugal pump through an outflow cannula, which is inserted into the femoral artery.

Offloading blood from the left atrium reduces the left ventricular preload and wall stress and, in turn, decreases the oxygen demand. Tandem Heart will increase the afterload, reduce the left ventricular stroke volume, reduce the left ventricular preload, and improve the peripheral tissue perfusion. (See Figure 4-9.)

Indications and Contraindications

The indications for Tandem Heart are generally the same indications as for Impella use. The main indications are refractory cardiogenic shock, high-risk PCI, myocarditis, percutaneous valve replacement, large myocardial infarction, and as a bridge to transplant.

Contraindications include severe peripheral vascular disease, sepsis, and irreversible neurologic disease. Other contraindications include ventricular septal defect, moderate to severe aortic regurgitations, and any contraindication for anticoagulation. In addition, the transseptal cannula set should not be used when any anatomic, medical, or physiologic impairment may harm the use of a femoral access procedure or transseptal access to the left atrium.

Equipment

Tandem Heart consists of 3 components:

1. Centrifugal pump
2. Arterial cannula
3. Transseptal cannula (has a curved tip with 14 side ports for drainage and is placed in left atrium)

Technique

- The first step is to prime the controller to make sure connections are ready, and tubing is carefully watched for air free connections.
- Femoral vein access is obtained using a 21-F cannula, and the device is secured over the wire in the left atrium by transseptal puncture.

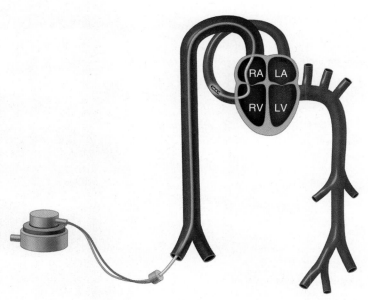

FIGURE 4-9. Configuration of Tandem Heart. LA, left atrium; LV, left ventricle; RA, right atrium; RV, right ventricle.

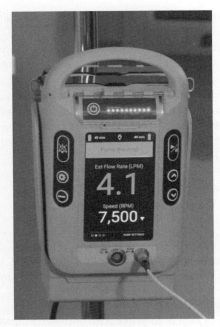

FIGURE 4-10. Interface of Tandem Heart.

- Two-staged dilator is used to implant device in left atrium.
- A 17-F arterial outflow cannula is inserted in the iliac artery via femoral artery.

- After de-airing the cannula, the connection is established with external pump.
- Anticoagulation is initiated with target activated clotting time (ACT) of 250 seconds.

Weaning From Tandem Heart

- After PCI is finished, the left atrium cannula can be withdrawn from IVC once ACT is 180 seconds, and the controller can be turned off at this point. The cannulas can then be withdrawn once ACT is less than 150 seconds and hemostasis can be achieved.
- For patients requiring long-term Tandem Heart use, an 8- to 14-hour weaning period is required. The pump speed is decreased by 0.5 L/min, and hemodynamics are carefully monitored. Once hemodynamics are improved, then cannula can be removed as outlined above.

Complications

Major complications of Tandem Heart are similar as IABP and Impella. Sepsis is reported to occur in about 30%, major bleeding is reported in 53% to 59%, hemolysis occurs in 5.3%, and limb ischemia is reported in 3% to 10% of cases.

It is important to note that major bleeding is more frequently experienced in patients undergoing Tandem Heart. This may be associated with the use of transseptal

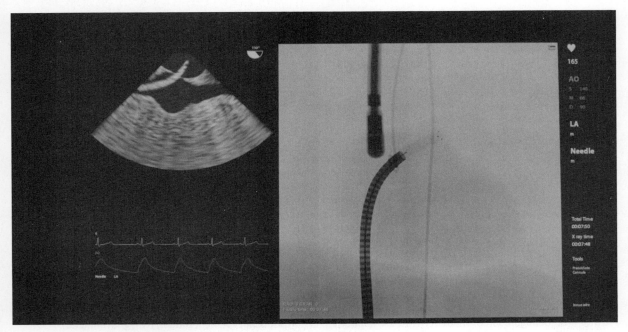

FIGURE 4-11. Placement of Tandem Heart cannula.

■ TABLE 4-5. Summary of Complications

Procedural Complications	Device-Related Complications
Bleeding	Device migration
Femoral arteriovenous fistula	Arial septal defect
Limb ischemia, wound infection, and lymphocele	Stroke

puncture, as well as the presence of 2 sites of percutaneous vascular access, with anticoagulation.

Other complications related to the Tandem Heart are dislodgement of inflow cannula and right to left shunt, which may lead to serious outcomes.

Troubleshooting

- The main issues that are encountered in Tandem Heart are related to catheter malposition or low flows.
- If the left atrial catheter is too deep, try to pull the catheter out slowly under transesophageal echocardiography or fluoroscopic guidance. If the blood in the catheter becomes darker, push it forward.
- In case of a low flow alarm, the main causes are inflow catheter malposition, dehydration, outflow catheter kink, or arterial stenosis.

Future Directions

- Tandem Heart is being explored for use in percutaneous aortic valve placement cases to provide hemodynamic support.
- Efforts are ongoing to improvise its use for RV support in RV or biventricular failure.

Percutaneous Right Ventricle Support Device

RV failure continues to be a major concern today. There are limited percutaneous MCS devices available with suboptimal efficiency. It depends on the algorithm of the devices available and the operator's experience. Currently, RV assist devices (RVADs) and surgically placed pumps are considered the preferred choice, and the percutaneous approach is still evolving.

Historical Perspective

Historically, RV support devices are surgically placed and can be used as extracorporeal centrifugal flow pumps. Use dates back to 1980, when surgically placed pulmonary artery (PA) balloon counterpulsation was used to support acute RV failure. This pump did not provide favorable RV hemodynamic outcomes and was replaced by rotary flow RVAD. The effort to improvise this concept to use it for a percutaneous approach was continued until 2019 when the FDA approved the Impella RP for select patients with cardiogenic shock secondary to RV failure. This helped in reducing the need for thoracotomy or open sternotomy. In 2014, the RECOVER-RIGHT trial showed improved mortality outcomes in 30 patients supported by Impella RP. Moreover, a similar concept was used to design a percutaneous RVAD called ProtekDuo to mitigate the invasive approach. This began another era of percutaneous RV devices with better cannulation size, approach, and pump algorithms. For the sake of convenience, we will discuss all RV devices together.

Mechanism of Action

The primary mechanism of action of both the Impella RP and ProtekDuo is similar in that both are meant to bypass the RV.

■ TABLE 4-6. Types of Right-Sided MCS

RV Support Devices	Access	Sheath Size	Pump	Flow (L/min)	Days
Impella RP	Femoral vein (connects IVC to PA)	22 F	Micro-axial	2-4	14
ProtekDuo with or without oxygenator	Internal jugular vein (2 lumens, single catheter) (connects right atrium to PA)	29 or 31 F	Centrifugal	4.5	
Venoarterial extracorporeal membrane oxygenation	Femoral vein and artery (bypass venous system)	18-21 F	Centrifugal	4-5	Weeks

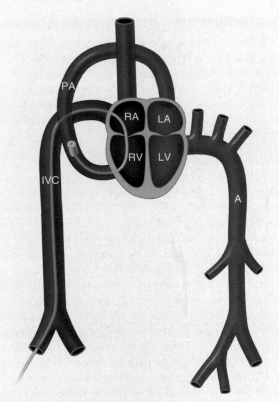

FIGURE 4-12. Configuration of Impella RP. A, aorta; IVC, inferior vena cava; LA, left atrium; LV, left ventricle; PA, pulmonary artery; RA, right atrium; RV, right ventricle.

Impella RP is a micro-axial pump that drains blood from the IVC and pumps it to the PA. The pump is inserted with venous access and advanced over a wire into the PA. The pump provides circulatory support for up to 14 days and is meant to deliver flow between 2 and 4 L/min. If combined with a left-sided Impella (described earlier), it provides biventricular support.

ProtekDuo with CentriMag is a special percutaneous RVAD designed as a single-access, double-lumen cannula placed in the internal jugular vein. It drains blood from the right atrium and pumps it to the PA using the same cannula. It can be used in different configurations to work as venovenous extracorporeal membrane oxygenation and helps in oxygenation. It can provide flow of about 4.5 L/min (See Figure 4-12).

Indications and Contraindications

RV support devices are indicated in cases where circulatory support is needed in patients with acute right heart failure after left ventricular assist device implantation, pulmonary hypertension crisis, heart transplant, bypass surgery, or biventricular failure after myocardial infarction. In general, placement of this device is contraindicated in cases of disorders of the PA structure that could interfere with proper positioning, severe tricuspid stenosis or regurgitation, severe pulmonic stenosis or regurgitation, mural thrombus, or presence of vena cava filter or caval interruption device. Any degree of anatomic disruption either from access point of view to advancement or placement will be a contraindication for the device. The ProtekDuo system has an added advantage of an internal jugular approach with more flow and patient ambulation.

Equipment

Impella RP consists of 2 components:

1. Catheter with inlet and outlet area along with differential pressure sensor
2. Automated controller for monitoring and controlling the catheter function

ProtekDuo and Tandem Heart consist of:

1. LIFESPARC pump: Powerful pump for blood flow
2. ProtekDuo Cannula: Novel double-lumen cannula with single access

Technique

- Femoral or internal jugular (for ProtekDuo) venous access is obtained using Seldinger technique.
- Flow-directed, balloon-tipped PA catheter is advanced to PA and then guidewire is inserted.
- Remove PA catheter and initiate anticoagulation with target ACT of 350 to 400 seconds.
- After sequential dilation, cannula can be inserted and wire removed with back end clamped.
- For ProtekDuo, distal port will be situated in main PA, and proximal port will be located in the right atrium. For clamping and bleed, proximal port will be used.
- For Impella RP, calibration can be done once cannula is in IVC. As the catheter exits the tricuspid valve, it needs to be torqued anteriorly. The desired course from tricuspid valve to PA should be straight without looping.
- Secure the cannula and prime the controller to make sure connections are ready and watch tubing carefully for air free connections.

Weaning

Impella weaning can be initiated once hemodynamic parameters are improving (including cardiac power

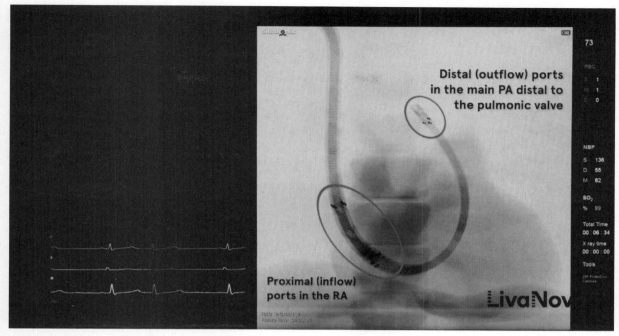

FIGURE 4-13. ProtekDuo under fluoroscopic view.

output, urine output, lactic acid, and pressor/inotropic requirement).

Once ready, Impella RP can be weaned down to a flow of 2 L/min and RV function reassessed. Once reassured, flow can be weaned to 0.5 L/min (P1 level), and cannula can be pulled to IVC. Remove the whole cannula once ACT is less than 150 seconds.

With ProtekDuo system, flow can be reduced to 2 L/min by gradual decrements of 0.5 L/min.

Hemostasis can be achieved by figure of 8/mattress suture.

Complications

In general, possible complications related to Impella RP/ProtekDuo placement are similar to those related to the regular Impella placement. These include bleeding, perforation, vascular complications, insertion site infection, cardiac arrhythmias, cardiac tamponade, hemolysis, hepatic failure, and tricuspid valve injury.

Troubleshooting

Many issues that may arise with Impella RP/ProtekDuo can be solved using the same troubleshooting steps described in the Impella and Tandem Heart sections.

For Impella RP, if it shows a low purge pressure, the first thing to do is to inspect the purge system for leaks. If there are no leaks, change to a purge fluid with a higher dextrose concentration. If the purge pressure is not stable, follow instructions on the device. However, if the alarm shows that the purge system is open, inspect the purge system for leaks. If no leaks are visible, the problem may be located at the level of the purge cassette.

It is also important to note that if the purge pressure exceeds 1100 mmHg, that is the time when the automated controller will display the low purge flow alarm. If the purge system is blocked, an alarm will be activated. At that time, the purge system needs to be checked, assessing for kinks or blockages; the concentration of dextrose in the purge solution needs to be decreased; and possibly, the purge system will need to be replaced.

In general, in case of low flow alarm, make sure the device position, catheter caliber, and patient hydration status are adequate.

Future Directions
- Efforts are ongoing to improve the algorithms on right-sided MCS devices.

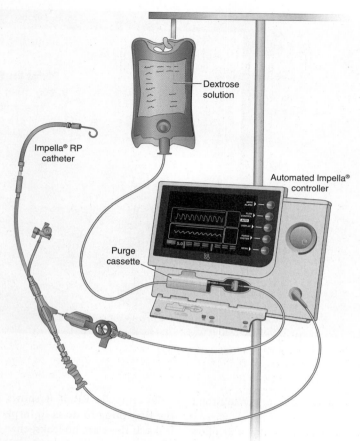

FIGURE 4-14. Impella RP configuration.

- Percutaneous devices are further improvised to improve flow demands and to mitigate the need for surgical RVAD placement.

SUGGESTED READINGS

Baldetti L, Beneduce A, Boccellino A, et al. Bedside intra-aortic balloon pump insertion in cardiac intensive care unit: a single-center experience. *Catheter Cardiovasc Interv.* 2022;99(7):1976-1983.

Francesca SL, Palanichamy N, Kar B, et al. First Use of the TandemHeart® Percutaneous Left Ventricular Assist Device as a Short-Term Bridge to Cardiac Transplantation. *Tex Heart Inst J.* 2006; 33(4): 490-491.

Hardy N, Starr N, Cosgrave J, Madhavan P. Intra-aortic balloon pump entrapment and surgical removal: a case report. *Eur Heart J Case Rep.* 2017;1(1):ytx002.

Impella Ventricular Support Systems for use during cardiogenic shock and high-risk PCI. Abiomed.

Impella RP with the automated Impella controller. Abiomed.

Kar B, Gregoric ID, Basra SS, et al. The percutaneous ventricular assist device in severe refractory cardiogenic shock. *J Am Coll Cardiol.* 2011;8;57(6):688-96.

Abbreviations

ACT: Activated clotting time
CAD: Coronary artery disease
ECG: Electrocardiogram
FDA: Food and Drug Administration
IABP: Intra-aortic balloon pump
IVC: Inferior vena cava
MCS: Mechanical circulatory support
PA: Pulmonary artery
PCI: Percutaneous coronary intervention
RV: Right ventricle
RVAD: Right ventricular assist device

CHAPTER 5

Durable Mechanical Circulatory Support

• *Nisha Ali, MD; Muhammad Saad, MD; Tamir D. Vittorio*

■ CASE PRESENTATION

A 35-year-old man presented to the emergency department with a chief complaint of progressive dyspnea, fatigue, and leg edema for past 2 weeks. He also reported a viral prodrome a few weeks ago. On arrival, he was found to be tachycardic and hypotensive. Patient denied any past medical or surgical history. He further denied any history of smoking, alcohol, or illicit drug use. The patient has no family history of cardiomyopathy.

The patient's transthoracic echocardiogram showed biventricular dysfunction with severely reduced left ventricular (LV) function of 10% with multiple LV thrombi. He was started on norepinephrine and inotropic support with dobutamine. He was also started on intravenous heparin for LV thrombus. He underwent invasive hemodynamics with right heart catheterization, which showed a pulmonary capillary wedge pressure of 25 mmHg, cardiac output of 4.4 CO Liter/min, and cardiac index of 2.0 CI L/min/m^2. Left heart catheterization showed patent coronaries. Cardiac magnetic resonance imaging showed mid-wall late gadolinium enhancement at basal interventricular septal segments. Broad-spectrum workup for dilated cardiomyopathy included normal thyroid function test, negative HIV panel, negative Lyme panel, negative antinuclear antibodies, and respiratory viral panel.

The patient's hospital course was complicated by progressive hypotension and tachycardia requiring intra-aortic balloon pump (IABP) placement. Despite being on an inotrope, vasopressor, and IABP, he remained tenuous and in a persistent low-output state refractory to medical treatment. He underwent left ventricular thrombectomy and implantation of an intracorporal LV assist device (LVAD; HeartMate 3). After LVAD implant, he continued to improve. Guideline-directed heart failure therapy was introduced, and he was eventually discharged in a stable condition.

■ KEY POINTS

- Durable mechanical circulatory support is used in advance heart failure management as a bridge to transplant, bridge to destination, and bridge to recovery.
- Several types of left, right, and biventricular devices are used to provide mechanical pumping to improve cardiac output.
- The HeartMate 3 device is the most common LVAD currently in use. These devices need to be meticulously managed and require frequent follow-up visits. They are associated with complications such as bleeding, infection, and strokes.
- Physical knowledge about these devices and their functions, mechanism, and complications is integral in optimizing these patients.

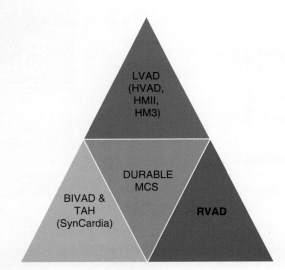

FIGURE 5-1. Types of durable MCS. BIVAD, biventricular assist device.

INTRODUCTION

Heart failure is one of the leading causes of morbidity and mortality worldwide. There are more than 6 million Americans living with heart failure with about 10% with advanced heart failure. Conventional heart failure therapies lead to improvement in left ventricular (LV) function in some patients, whereas in other patients, there is a progressive worsening of symptoms and cardiac function, leading to advanced chronic heart failure. These patients continue to remain symptomatic even at rest,

have frequent hospitalizations due to decompensation, and have overall poor prognosis. Guideline-directed medical and device-based therapies are no longer effective in improving symptoms and cardiac function, and these patients need advanced heart failure therapies with a durable mechanical circulatory support device and heart transplant. Some patients might even need palliative care.

These patients cannot be classified using the New York Heart Association (NYHA) classification due to complexity of symptoms. Hence, the Interagency Registry for Mechanically Assisted Circulatory Support (INTERMACS) classification was developed (Figure 5-1). This classification stratifies patients into 7 clinical profiles to describe the severity of their heart failure (Table 5-1).

■ DURABLE MECHANICAL CIRCULATORY SUPPORT DEVICE

In patients with advanced heart failure that is refractory to guideline-directed medical or device therapy, mechanical circulatory support (MCS) with either a ventricular assist device (VAD) or artificial heart is needed for symptom relief and to improve survival and quality of life. Patients with durable MCS require frequent follow-up, self-care for management of their device, and awareness of its complications.

Candidates for Durable Mechanical Circulatory Support

Table 5-2 lists the indications for MCS.

■ TABLE 5-1. INTERMACS Classification		
Profile	Characteristics	Description
INTERMACS 1	Cardiogenic shock	Life-threating hypotension despite escalating intravenous ionotropic support
INTERMACS 2	Progressive decline	Progressive decline on intravenous ionotropic support
INTERMACS 3	Stable but inotrope dependent	Stable on continuous intravenous ionotropic support
INTERMACS 4	Resting symptoms	Daily symptoms of congestion at rest or during activities of daily living
INTERMACS 5	Exertion intolerant	Comfortable at rest and activities of daily living but cannot engage in activities above that
INTERMACS 6	Exertion limited	Participates in minor activity but fatigues quickly
INTERMACS 7	Advanced NYHA class III	Comfortable with meaningful activity, limited to mild exertion

Source: Adapted from Stevenson LW, Pagani FD, Young JB, et al. INTERMACS profiles of advanced heart failure: the current picture. J Heart Lung Transplant. 2009;28(6):535-541.

<table>
<tr><td>■ TABLE 5-2. Indication of Durable MCS</td></tr>
</table>

Advance heart failure requiring frequent hospitalizations
NYHA class IV symptoms despite being on guideline-
  directed medical therapy
Intolerance to neurohormonal antagonist
Increased requirements for or refractory to diuretics
Signs of end organ dysfunction secondary to low cardiac
  output
Inotrope dependent
Low peak VO_2(<12 mL/kg/min)
Refractory ventricular arrhythmias

Types of Durable Mechanical Circulatory Devices

VAD and artificial heart are the 2 most common devices used in patients with advanced refractory heart failure, with VAD being most frequently used. Several factors need to be considered when deciding which device is appropriate for the patient.

Assessment Before Mechanical Circulatory Device Placement

Right Heart Dysfunction Right ventricular (RV) failure is one of the most common causes of morbidity and mortality in patients with LV assist device (LVAD). Patients should have detailed RV function assessment prior to LVAD placement.

The following parameters lead to increased risk of RV failure:

- Central venous filling pressure (CVP) ≥15 mmHg
- RV stroke work index <0.5 mmHg × L/m²
- Pulmonary artery pressure index <2.0
- Pulmonary capillary wedge pressure to central venous pressure ratio >0.63
- Signs of liver congestion and coagulopathy, moderate to severe tricuspid regurgitation, and tricuspid annular plane systolic excursion <1.4 cm/s

Valve Dysfunction Abnormal valve function can increase the risk of LVAD implantation. Normal or near-normal function of aortic valve is required for proper LV unloading. Tricuspid valve regurgitation might need repair at the time of LVAD implant due to risk of future RV failure. Mitral stenosis needs to be corrected at the time of implant because the left atrium needs to unload blood to the left ventricle. A prosthetic valve can increase the risk of stroke. A mechanical aortic valve is an absolute contraindication to LVAD unless it is replaced with a bioprosthetic valve.

Stroke Risk Stroke is one of the complications of MCS. Patients undergoing LVAD need complete evaluation including neurologic and peripheral vascular disease assessment. This includes computed tomography (CT) of the head, ultrasound of carotids, lower extremity ultrasound, and ankle-brachial index measurement.

Great Vessel Calcification CT of the chest is required to assess aorta and to look for calcification because its presence is a contraindication since device requires anastomosis to the aorta.

Noncardiovascular Assessment

- Pulmonary function test and CT chest are required for assessment of pulmonary function because decreased function increases perioperative morbidity and mortality. Contraindications to VAD placement include decreased exercise capacity secondary to lung condition, dependence on supplemental oxygen, and decreased forced expiratory volume in 1 second less than 1 L or diffusing capacity for carbon monoxide less than 25% of predicted that is not attributable to heart failure.
- Ultrasound or CT of abdomen is needed to assess liver function because liver cirrhosis and fibrosis with signs of liver dysfunction are contraindications for MCS device implantation.
- Kidney injury has been associated with MCS. Patients with underlying kidney dysfunction, including patients on hemodialysis, are at increased risk for infection and bleeding and are difficult to manage. MCS is typically contraindicated in patients with severe kidney dysfunction who have low probability of renal recovery and require hemodialysis.
- Patients with MCS require lifelong anticoagulation. Preoperative bleeding risk assessment is required because severe anemia, thrombocytopenia, bleeding diathesis, and warfarin intolerance are some of the contraindications for MCS placement.

■ LEFT VENTRICLE ASSISTED DEVICE

LVAD is the device of choice in patients with predominant left heart failure with reduced LV function. It has a tendency to flow about 10 L/min of blood and has been associated with improved survival in advanced heart failure patients. Currently, LVAD is being used in heart failure patients awaiting transplantation.

■ **TABLE 5-3.** Various Classes of LVAD

	XVE (First Generation)	HMII (Second Generation)	HVAD (Third Generation)	HM3 (Third Generation)
Technology	Piston and cylinder model	Archimede's screw model	Hydrodynamic levitation	Electromagnetic levitation
Location	Extracorporeal	Intraperitoneal	Intrapericardial	Intrapericardial
Flow	Pulsatile	Axial (continuous)	Centrifugal (continuous)	Centrifugal (continuous)
Goals of care	BTT and DT	BTT, DT, and BTC	BTT, DT, and BTC	BTT, DT, and BTC
Pros	Mimics cardiac contractility (obsolete)	First MCS approved	Small, good battery life, no mechanical friction points	Small, good battery life, no levitation speed required, wider gaps to avoid RBC trauma
Cons	Noisier, mechanical failure	Large size	Critical speed required to reach rotor levitation	More data required.

Abbreviations: BTC, bridge to candidacy; BTT, bridge to transplantation; DT, destination therapy; RBC, red blood cell.

Types of LVAD

The 3 most commonly used LVADs are listed below. In addition, first-generation LVADs are listed in Table 5-3.

- HeartMate II (HMII; Abbott Laboratories, Abbott Park, Illinois)
- HeartMate 3 (HM3; Abbott Laboratories, Abbott Park, Illinois)
- HeartWare Ventricular Assist Device (HVAD; Medtronic, Minneapolis, Minnesota)

Historical Background

VAD was approved by the US Food and Drug Administration (FDA) in 1994 as a pulsatile pump (HeartMate XVE) with bridge to transplantation. With its intricate design and variety, it showed great improvement in quality of life and survival rate (52% vs 25% with medical management) but at the cost of numerous neurologic and bleeding complications. This led to the introduction of a new generation of continuous flow pumps with smaller size and improved flow with less risk of pump thrombosis and lower complication rate. This was shown in 2007 in

the Bridge to Transplant trial and in 2009 in the Destination Therapy trial, with additional survival up to 70% with HMII and HVAD compared to HeartMate XVE.

Furthermore, with improved technology of centrifugal flow, randomized controlled trials continued to show increased long-term survival. Recently, in the MOMENTUM 3 trial, 1020 patients were randomized 1:1 to receive either the HM3 or HMII device. The trial showed improved 6-month survival in the HM3 group with less risk of pump malfunction and thrombosis. In 2021, HVAD was taken off the market due to increased risk of neurologic events and increased mortality. Currently, HM3 is the most commonly implanted LVAD available on the market.

Mechanism of Action

LVAD is a surgically (via sternotomy or robotic-assisted) implanted electromechanical pump that augments pumping of the heart. It supports patients by increasing cardiac output, increasing perfusion, and decreasing filling pressure of the failing ventricle. It consists of 4 parameters including speed, flow, power, and pulsatility index (Table 5-4).

■ **TABLE 5-4.** LVAD Parameters

Parameters	Mechanism	HMII	HM3	HVAD
Speed (rpm)	Higher speed more unloading	8000-10,000	5000-6000	2400-3200
Flow (L/min)	Estimated value	4-6	4-6	4-6
Power (watts)	Directly related to speed and volume	5-8	4-7	3-7
Pulsatility index	Reflects native contractility	5-8	3-5	2-4

- Speed is primarily set by the clinician and is the tendency to unload the LV. It tracks the pulsatility and drops to a lower speed limit to avoid suction events. Higher speed will cause less mitral regurgitation and less aortic valve opening. Artificial pulse (in HM3) or Lavare cycle (in HVAD) is the fluctuation in speed to avoid blood stasis and pump thrombosis.
- Power is the amount of energy needed to maintain the speed.
- Flow (in liters per minute) is the estimated calculation based on pump speed, power consumption, and pressure difference between the cannula. It takes hematocrit into account for calculation in centrifugal pumps.
- Pulsatility index is the inherent ability of the LV contractility and is related to speed.

Indications and Contraindications

Patient selection is an important step in LVAD implantation. Careful review of medication adherence, support system, and hemodynamic parameters should be performed. Shared decision making is required to achieve realistic goals with patients and caregivers (Table 5-5).

- Bridge to transplantation: In patients who are eligible and awaiting cardiac transplantation, the MCS device can be used as a bridge to transplantation.
- Bridge to candidacy or bridge to decision: LVAD can be implanted to clarify candidacy prior to transplantation. It is generally reserved for patients who have contraindications for heart transplant, such as substance use disorder or renal dysfunction, who need further management before decision for heart transplant.

■ **TABLE 5-5. CMS Criteria for LVAD Selection**

NYHA class IV
LV ejection fraction <25%
Inotrope dependent
Cardiac index <2.2 if not on inotropes with failed GDMT for 2 months or advanced HF for 14 days on temporary MCS
Low-sodium, high-diuretic need, high-risk cardiopulmonary exercise test findings, poor tolerance of GDMT, refractory VT/VF

Abbreviations: CMS, Centers for Medicare and Medicaid Services; GDMT, guideline-directed medical therapy; HF, heart failure; VF, ventricular fibrillation; VT, ventricular tachycardia.

- Destination therapy: Patients who are not candidates for heart transplant or any other long-term therapy may undergo MCS as destination therapy.
- Bridge to recovery: In very few cases, MCS can be used as a bridge to recovery, such as in patients with myocarditis or after myocardial infarction.

When considering referral for LVAD, one should think about the operative risk for LVAD and risk of death with medical management of heart failure. A multidisciplinary discussion should be conducted to decide the candidacy for LVAD. LVAD is generally avoided in the following conditions:

- Irreversible renal, hepatic, or neurologic disorder
- Metastatic cancer
- Irreversible coagulation and bleeding disorder
- Medication nonadherence and substance dependence
- Psychosocial limitation
- Severe RV failure
- Active systemic infection

■ **TABLE 5-6. HFSA Guideline for Durable MCS**

Recommendation	COR	LOE
In select patients with advanced HFrEF with NYHA class IV symptoms who are deemed to be dependent on continuous intravenous inotropes or temporary MCS, durable LVAD implantation is effective to improve functional status, QOL, and survival.	1	A
In select patients with advanced HFrEF who have NYHA class IV symptoms despite GDMT, durable MCS can be beneficial to improve symptoms, improve functional class, and reduce mortality.	2a	B-R
In patients with advanced HFrEF and hemodynamic compromise and shock, temporary MCS, including percutaneous and extracorporeal ventricular assist devices, are reasonable as a "bridge to recovery" or "bridge to decision."	2a	B-NR

Abbreviations: COR, class of recommendation; GDMT, guideline-directed medical therapy; HFrEF, heart failure with reduced ejection fraction; HFSA, Heart Failure Society of America; LOE, level of evidence; QOL, quality of life.

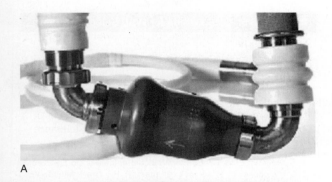

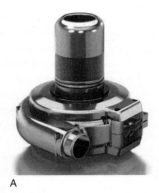

A

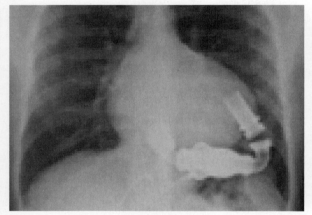

B

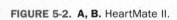

FIGURE 5-2. A, B. HeartMate II.

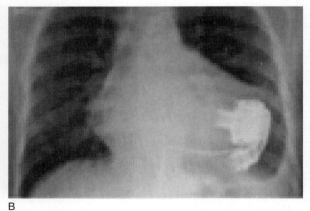

B

FIGURE 5-3. A, B. HeartMate 3.

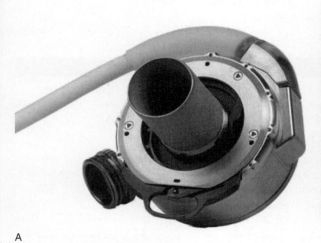

A

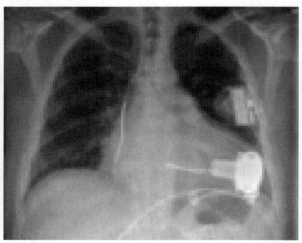

B

FIGURE 5-4. A, B. HVAD.

Equipment

LVAD consists of an inflow cannula, outflow cannula, continuous flow pump, driveline, and an electrical controller.

- Inflow cannula is a metal tube that is inserted to the apex of left ventricle and directs blood from left ventricle to the pump.
- Impeller sits in a titanium pump that speeds the blood and sends it to the aorta.
- Outflow cannula is connected to the synthetic graft and is attached to the ascending aorta.
- Driveline is electrical wiring that is tunneled via abdominal wall and is connected to the power source, such as batteries and external controller.

Postimplant Care

- Initiation of antiplatelet therapy and anticoagulation should be considered as soon as postoperative hemostasis is achieved.
- Aspirin can be initiated in a low dose around postoperative day 2.
- Heparin can be started once appropriate before initiation of warfarin at low target rate and then switched to warfarin with goal international normalized ratio (INR) of 2 to 3.
- Blood pressure should be monitored and controlled at a target mean arterial pressure between 70 and 80 mmHg.

- All patients should be monitored for early or late right heart failure by assessment of hemodynamics and clinical features.

Blood Pressure Monitoring in LVAD Patients

- Continuous-flow LVAD has narrow pulse pressure, and it is difficult to assess blood pressure in these patients by automated blood pressure monitor.
- Therefore, Doppler probe can be used to assess antecubital brachial artery pressure, reflecting systolic blood pressure.
- Palpation and auscultation methods cannot be used in continuous-flow LVAD to assess blood pressure.

Role of Echocardiography in LVAD Management

- Echocardiography is used to assess suitability for LVAD candidacy. Cavity size can be assessed for LVAD consideration because a less dilated LV (<6.3 cm) may not benefit from implant.
- Evaluation of LV thrombus, intracardiac shunts, LV ejection fraction, and valvular disease (greater than mild mitral stenosis, mechanical valves, and aortic regurgitation) should be performed.
- Evaluation of RV function is a key assessment before LVAD implant that can impact decision making. RV dimensions by echocardiography, including size,

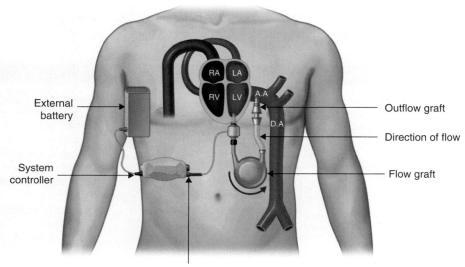

FIGURE 5-5. LVAD configuration. (See color insert.)

systolic function, and degree of tricuspid regurgitation, should be assessed.

- After implant, surveillance echocardiogram is needed to assess the device function and hemodynamic response. Optimization of LVAD speed can by assessed by LV geometry, septum position, opening of aortic valve, and degree of mitral regurgitation.
- In case of LVAD alarm troubleshooting, bedside echocardiogram can be used to assess inferior vena cava size, RV function, tamponade, and device position to guide further management.

Troubleshooting LVAD Alarms (Table 5-7)

- Optimal speed of LVAD consists of minimizing mitral regurgitation and allowing aortic valve to open 2 to 3 times per cycle with maximum RV function. A speed that is too low results in suboptimal LV unloading, less aortic valve opening, and risk of pump thrombosis.
- Power is dependent on volume, and vasodilation such as sepsis or aortic regurgitation increases the power usage. Pump thrombosis also increases power usage. In contrast, conditions such as inflow cannula stenosis/malposition and pannus decrease power usage. Hypertension and outflow cannula obstruction can also lead to more power usage.
- Flow and power are used interchangeably during troubleshooting LVAD alarms.

Complications of LVADs

Bleeding: Patients with continuous-flow LVAD are at higher risk of bleeding events secondary to microvascular

dysfunction, angiodysplasia, and neurohormonal imbalances. Bleeding in the first few days after implantation is mostly surgery related. Bleeding that occurs later in the course includes gastrointestinal bleeding from arteriovenous malformation or acquired von Willebrand syndrome (due to sheered hemolysis). Intracranial bleeding is another important site. In the Destination Therapy trial, there was an 11% risk of hemorrhagic stroke in the first 2 years after LVAD (HMII) placement.

Thrombosis: Patients with LVAD are at increased risk for stroke, transient ischemic attack, arterial thrombosis, and pump thrombosis despite being on antiplatelet and anticoagulant therapy, and these are often the primary cause of death. Pump thrombosis can cause device malfunction and embolic strokes. Pump thrombosis can be diagnosed by evidence of hemolysis, heart failure symptoms, increase in device power, and device alarms. Uncontrolled blood pressure, suboptimal anticoagulation, lower speed, and suboptimal position of pump are a few factors directly related to thrombosis risk. Treatment is additional anticoagulation and fibrinolytics.

Infections: Infections are a common cause of morbidity and the leading cause of readmission among LVAD patients, especially after 3 months of implant. Data from the INTERMACS registry indicated that pneumonia and sepsis are the most common infectious complications in patients with LVADs (23% and 20%, respectively), followed by driveline site infections, which occur in approximately 19% of patients within 1 year after implant. Non-VAD infections such as endocarditis, catheter-related bloodstream infections, and mediastinitis are also common in VAD patients.

Power	PI	Alarm	Causes	Management
Low	Low	Low flow alarm	Hypovolemia, bleeding, tamponade, right heart failure, and outflow graft thrombosis/kink	Check CBC, INR, ECG, and CXR and assess volume status, IV fluids, TTE (if needed)
Low	High	Low flow alarm	Hypertension Low speed Inflow/outflow obstruction	Control blood pressure; if still persistent, consider imaging
High	Low	High flow alarm	Hypotension, sepsis, high speed, pump thrombosis, significant AR	Hydration and inotropes
High	High	No alarm	Exercise Improvement in native function	Reassurance

■ TABLE 5-7. LVAD Troubleshooting

Abbreviations: AR, aortic regurgitation; CBC, complete blood count; CXR, chest X-ray; ECG, electrocardiogram; IV, intravenous; PI, XXXX; TTE, transthoracic echocardiography.

■ TABLE 5-8. Long-Term Complications of LVAD

Complication	Cause	Diagnosis	Treatment
Bleeding (most commonly gastrointestinal bleed)	Arteriovenous malformations, hemolysis	Clinical history, endoscopy, capsule endoscopy, CT angiography, or nuclear tagged RBC scan	Resuscitation, transfusion, anticoagulation interruption briefly, endoscopic interventions such as clipping, epinephrine injection, heater probe
CVA (ischemic and hemorrhagic)	Poor BP control, suboptimal anticoagulation, atrial fibrillation	Clinical exam, CT/MRI brain	Appropriate use of antiplatelet therapy and anticoagulation, optimize BP control
Pump thrombosis	Lower pump speed, suboptimal anticoagulation, and device malposition	Hemolysis, new heart failure symptoms and device alarms, CT angiography, TTE and cardiac catheterization	BP control, anticoagulation, mechanical support, and fibrinolytics (replacement if needed)
Infection	Device contamination with skin flora	Clinical exam or imaging, if needed	Antibiotics, debridement (driveline site), or chronic suppressive therapy
Arrhythmia	Suction events, electrolyte imbalance	Clinical, telemonitor	Antiarrhythmic agents, catheter ablation
RV failure	Increase preload, change in LV geometry	Clinical findings and elevated CVP (>16 mmHg) with worsening symptoms of right heart failure	Mechanical support

Abbreviations: BP, blood pressure; CVA, cerebrovascular accident; MRI, magnetic resonance imaging; RBC, red blood cell; TTE, transthoracic echocardiography.

RV failure: RV failure is one of the most common causes of morbidity and mortality in VAD patients and occurs in approximately 11% of patients with LVAD. RV dysfunction can result from increased preload from higher cardiac output from LV, increased afterload from pulmonary hypertension, and septal shift from left to right due to increased pump speed. Diagnosis should be made early based on evidence of higher CVP and its clinical manifestations (eg, ascites, renal or liver failure). Inotropic support or mechanical support is often required in management of RV failure.

Aortic insufficiency: Aortic insufficiency occurs in some patients with LVAD. Mechanisms include pressure in aortic root, variable blood flow, and incorrect angle between outflow graft and aorta. It is diagnosed by surveillance echocardiogram and may require surgical intervention if clinically severe.

Future Directions

- Advanced engineering technology is being used to improve pump design/size and battery longevity. Drivelines are hypothesized to be fully contained rather externalized.
- Better surgical techniques including minimally invasive technology are under consideration.
- Outcome scores for predicting RV failure in LVAD patients are being formulated to improve survival after LVAD implant.

■ RIGHT VENTRICULAR ASSIST DEVICE

- RV assist devices (RVADs) can be used in patients with predominant right-sided heart failure. Placement of isolated RVAD is rare, and its long-term efficacy is not very well known.

- RV failure after LVAD implantation is associated with increased morbidity and mortality. It can occur either perioperatively or postoperatively.
- Some of the reasons include surgical stress, pulmonary hypertension, and increased RV preload secondary to near normalization of cardiac output.
- Temporary percutaneous RVADs have been used increasingly in patients undergoing LVAD placement with risk of RV failure.
- RV function often improves eventually with successful device removal. RVAD has been discussed in detail elsewhere.

■ BIVENTRICULAR ASSIST DEVICE

In patients with biventricular systolic or diastolic dysfunction, biventricular assist devices in the form of either LVAD with temporary RVAD configuration or a total artificial heart are being used. The devices can only be used as a bridge to transplant.

■ ARTIFICIAL HEART

Total artificial heart (TAH) is another form of MCS used in patients with end-stage biventricular dysfunction as a bridge to transplantation. It is also used in patients in whom LVAD cannot be placed due to an anatomic barrier. TAH is implanted in a much smaller subset of patients as compared to LVAD, and only 44 patients are alive on this device globally as of 2020. The surgery is performed in very limited centers across the world.

Historical Background

The first permanent artificial heart, Jarvik 7, was implanted by Dr. Robert Jarvik in 1982. It consisted of 2 air-powered pumps that pushed blood through the valves using drivelines. It required a larger console for power control and was ultimately taken off the market. Later, it was introduced as CardioWest Total Artificial Heart, which received FDA approval. This device was renamed in 2010 as SynCardia temporary, which showed promising survival benefits in patients waiting for transplantation. In March 2010, SynCardia released Freedom Driver, which replaced the large pneumatic console of TAH and has emerged as a game changer. With this innovation, the patient does not need to be in hospital awaiting transplant. Currently, the 70 cc SynCardia (SynCardia Systems, Tucson, Arizona) is the most commonly implanted TAH and has an extremely high cost.

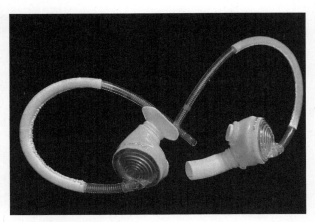

FIGURE 5-6. SynCardia. (See color insert).

Mechanism of Action

TAH is a pulsatile pump capable of pumping 9 L/min of blood. A TAH consists of pneumatically driven pumps that replace both ventricles, all valves, and the proximal portion of the great vessels.

The valves are replaced by 2 tilting disk mechanical valves, and flow is generated by a pneumatically driven diaphragm. The driver controls the air flow via driveline and helps in pumping blood like a piston model.

Device Parameters

- Ejection rate: Equivalent to pump beat rate
- Drive pressure: Equivalent to contractility
- Time in systole: Equivalent to ejection time
- Vacuum pressure: Equivalent to filling pressure

Indications

Patients with advanced biventricular heart failure and shock in whom RV recovery is not expected are candidates for TAH. In addition, patients who are post myocardial infarction with ventricular septal defect, aortic dissection, cardiac graft failure, LV thrombus, refractory arrhythmia, or restrictive/infiltrative cardiomyopathy and who may not be candidates for LVAD can get TAH.

Contraindications

Patients who are not candidates for transplantation cannot receive TAH. Patients on anticoagulation or with smaller body size (body surface area <1.7m^2) or smaller chest cavity are also not the candidates for TAH.

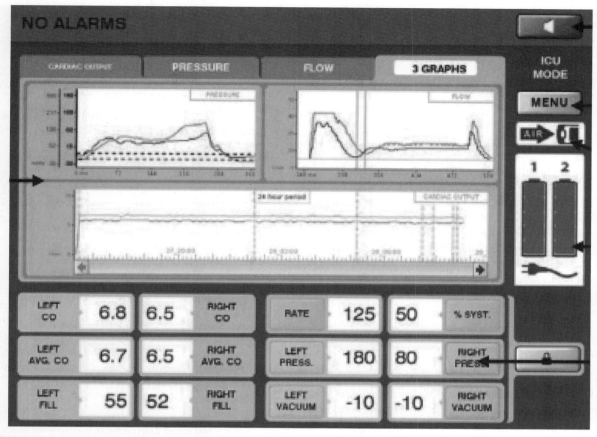

FIGURE 5-7. TAH interface. (See color insert.)

Equipment

TAH consists of the following parts:

- Mechanical pump that replaces patients' native ventricles and valve. The pump works on the principle of fully eject (prevent stasis) and partially fill (to allow reserve volume). Cannula and drivelines: Synthetic tubing connecting pump with driver.
- External driver placed outside the body that controls the pump. Beat-to-beat ejection pressure and airflow velocity are displayed on the console.

Troubleshooting

- Hypertension and volume management can address major issues in TAH troubleshooting.
- To optimize cardiac output, pump beat rate, drive pressure, percent time in systole, and vacuum pressure can be adjusted.

- Loss of eject waveform signifies high filling volume, and fluid overload/hypertension should be treated.
- Low fill volume warrants evaluation for hypovolemia, tamponade, and inflow obstruction.
- Anticoagulation with warfarin (INR 2.5-3.0) or aspirin is essential to mitigate thrombotic risk guided by thromboelastography.
- Portable drivers are afterload sensitive and need optimum blood pressure control for functioning.

Complications of TAH (Table 5-9)

- The major complications of TAH include bleeding, infection, and stroke.
- The lungs and the urinary tract system are the most common sites of infection.
- Postprocedure oliguric renal failure is a frequent complication. Severe renal dysfunction with rise in serum

■ TABLE 5-9. TAH Complications	
MCS-Related Complications	TAH Unique Complications
Infection/sepsis	Renal failure
Bleeding	Chronic anemia
Ischemic/hemorrhagic stroke	
Device malfunction	

creatinine and need for dialysis is seen postoperatively in up to 12% of patients.

- It has been postulated that interruption of neurohormonal compensatory mechanisms due to loss of natriuretic peptides may precipitate renal failure. Patients who do develop oliguric renal failure have a prompt and robust increase in urine output following nesiritide infusion without worsening of hemodynamics.
- Anemia due to hemolysis and ineffective erythropoiesis is another common complication associated with TAH, which may ultimately improve after transplantation.

Future Directions

- Use of TAH as destination therapy is under evaluation.
- Attempts to improve sizing of device for small thoracic spaces are ongoing with better troubleshooting algorithms.

SUGGESTED READINGS

Copeland JG, Smith RG, Arabia FA, et al. Total artificial heart bridge to transplantation: a 9-year experience with 62 patients. *J Heart Lung Transplant*. 2004;23:823-831.

Delgado R 3rd, Wadia Y, Kar B, et al. Role of B-type natriuretic peptide and effect of nesiritide after total cardiac replacement with the AbioCor total artificial heart. *J Heart Lung Transplant*. 2005;24:1166-1170.

Kirklin JK, Naftel DC, Pagani FD, et al. Seventh INTERMACS annual report: 15,000 patients and counting. *J Heart Lung Transplant*. 2015;34(12):1495-1504.

Stevenson LW, Pagani FD, Young JB, et al. INTERMACS profiles of advanced heart failure: the current picture. *J Heart Lung Transplant*. 2009;28(6):535-541.

Abbreviations

CT: Computed tomography
CVP: Central venous pressure
FDA: Food and Drug Administration
HM3: HeartMate 3
HMII: HeartMate II
HVAD: HeartWare Ventricular Assist Device
IABP: Intra-aortic balloon pump
INR: International normalized ratio
INTERMACS: Interagency Registry for Mechanically Assisted Circulatory Support
LV: Left ventricular
LVAD: Left ventricular assist device
MCS: Mechanical circulatory support
NYHA: New York Heart Association
RV: Right ventricular
RVAD: Right ventricular assist device
TAH: Total artificial heart
VAD: Ventricular assist device

CHAPTER 6

Fluid Management, Hemodynamic Assessment, and Fluid Removal Devices

• Shoaib Ashraf, MD; Muhammad Saad, MD; Muhammad Hassan, MD

■ CASE PRESENTATION

A 44-year-old woman with a past medical history of hypertension, renal artery stenosis, blood loss anemia from menorrhagia, and idiopathic pulmonary arterial hypertension (PAH) came to the hospital for right heart catheterization (RHC). She was diagnosed with PAH 12 years ago when she was worked up for systemic hypertension. She was found to have systolic pulmonary arterial pressure of 150 mmHg and elevated pulmonary vascular resistance (PVR) of 15 Wood units. Follow-up RHC 4 months ago showed mean pulmonary artery pressure (mPAP) of 53 mmHg and PVR of 18 Wood units. She was on bosentan 125 mg every 12 hours, sildenafil citrate 40 mg every 8 hours, and selexipag 1600 µg every 12 hours. Repeat RHC now showed mPAP of 48 mmHg and PVR of 12 Wood units. After discussion with the patient, the decision was made to titrate down selexipag, switch her to the up-titrating dose of intravenous treprostinil, keep the right heart catheter in place to guide the right dose, and monitor pulmonary artery pressures and other hemodynamic variables. This case shows the importance of RHC in the evaluation and differential diagnosis of pulmonary hypertension and assessment of response to therapies.

■ KEY POINTS

- Fluid assessment in critically ill patients is the key to improve short- and long-term outcomes.
- Invasive and noninvasive modalities are available to guide the fluid assessment and responsiveness of hemodynamically unstable patients.
- All information should be used in clinical context to obtain optimal results.

■ INTRODUCTION

Fluid assessment in the critical care unit is an important measure to guide management and improve patient outcomes. Current techniques use pressure and volume to estimate fluid status. Various methods have been proposed to provide effective assessment tools, but none of them is specific. Good judgment is required to incorporate the findings into the clinical scenario.

■ TABLE 6-1. Invasive Versus Noninvasive Devices	
Invasive	**Noninvasive**
Central venous catheter	Point-of-care ultrasound
Pulmonary artery catheter	Focused cardiac ultrasound
Left ventricle end-diastolic pressure (LVEDP)	Pulse pressure variation
	Doppler waveform
	Near-infrared spectroscopy

■ CENTRAL VENOUS CATHETER

Central venous catheter (CVC) is an invasive tool traditionally used to care for critically ill patients. Besides measuring central venous pressure (CVP), a pressure in the thoracic vena cava (TVC) near the right atrium, CVC can also help with administering peripherally incompatible infusions, placing devices, parenteral nutrition, and blood sampling.

Mechanism of Action

A normal CVP ranges between 3 and 8 mmHg, which can fluctuate depending on the patient's volume status and venous compliance. CVP is an important factor in critical care because it enables estimation of volume status and right ventricle (RV) function and assessment of cardiac

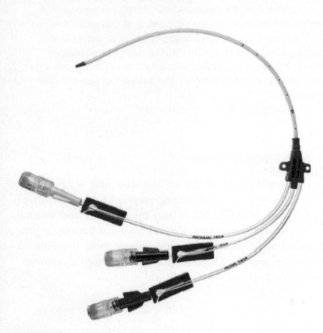

FIGURE 6-1. CVC catheter.

function via mixed venous gas. However, there are drawbacks and complications with CVC.

Indications

There are several indications for CVC placement.

- Hemodynamic monitoring, including measuring CVP and central venous oxygen saturation and assessing RV function in managing heart failure, critical care, perioperative, and septic patients
- Multiple peripherally incompatible infusions, including vasopressors, hyperosmolar solutions, chemotherapeutic drugs, and total parenteral nutrition
- The need for extracorporeal therapies, such as extracorporeal membrane oxygenation, hemodialysis, hemofiltration, and plasmapheresis
- For several venous interventions and medical devices, including placement of inferior vena cava filter, pulmonary artery catheter (PAC), interventional thrombolytic therapies, and transvenous cardiac pacemakers/defibrillators

Contraindications

Relative and site-specific absolute contraindications include the following:

- Skin or soft tissue infection
- Traumatic vascular injury proximal to the site of the catheter insertion
- Anatomic occlusion due to a thrombus, congenital anomalies, or another indwelling intravascular hardware
- Severe thrombocytopenia (platelet count $<20 \times 10^9$/L), which seems to have a higher probability of adverse events
- Severe coagulopathy with international normalized ratio (INR) greater than 3, although the actual incidence of major bleeding is less than 1%
- Agitated, uncooperative patient

Complications

Many potential complications can occur during the placement of CVC or after the procedure, including the following:

- External or internal bleeding in a coagulopathic patient
- Arterial puncture, arteriovenous fistula, or pseudoaneurysm
- Cardiac injury and pericardial effusion

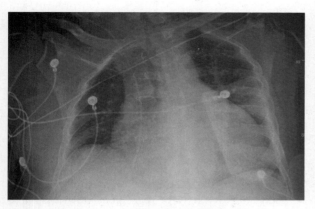

FIGURE 6-2. Chest radiograph showing central line.

- Hematoma formation leading to airway obstruction
- Pneumothorax from lung puncture
- Arrhythmias from irritation of the ventricles or atria by a guidewire
- Catheter-related bloodstream infections and exit site infection
- Central vein obstruction
- Venous air embolism
- Catheter-related deep venous thrombosis
- Catheter malfunction due to mechanical obstruction
- Embolization/migration of catheter components

Troubleshooting

- The CVC should be zeroed and referenced before taking readings.
- The patient should preferably lie in the supine position or approximately at a 30-degree angle in a semi-recumbent position.
- Under- or overdamped waveform: Underdamping is caused by excessive tubing lengths, high-output states, or tachycardia. An overdamped waveform occurs due to air bubbles in the tubing, a kinked catheter, or when the catheter tip becomes partially occluded by the blood clot or vessel wall. These factors should be systematically addressed.

■ PULMONARY ARTERY CATHETER

Introduction

A pulmonary artery catheter (PAC) or Swan-Ganz catheter is a 5-port balloon-tipped catheter placed into a pulmonary artery that can be used to evaluate and manage numerous cardiovascular conditions. It is named after its inventors, Jeremy Swan and William Ganz. The catheter is introduced through a central vein, after which the balloon is inflated, and it floats through the TVC to the right atrium and RV, and from there, the catheter is advanced to the pulmonary artery to obtain pulmonary capillary occlusive pressure (PCOP). Insertion and advancement of PAC can be monitored by a distinctive pattern of pressure waveform seen on the monitor, which helps determine the place of the catheter tips. Alternatively, the PAC can be placed in the catheterization lab under fluoroscopic guidance and the catheter tip maneuvered in the desired direction. PAC provides multiple direct and indirect measurements of hemodynamic variables.

Mechanism of Action

Accurately placed PAC helps directly measure the following hemodynamic variables.

- TVC pressure and CVP
- Central venous oxygen saturation for suspected shunt
- Right atrial pressure (RAP)
- RV pressure
- Pulmonary arterial pressure (PAP)
- Pulmonary capillary occlusion/wedge pressure
- Mixed venous oxygen saturation
- Thermodilution cardiac output (CO)
- Pulmonary artery wedge oxygen saturation

Many hemodynamic variables can be derived from the measurements mentioned earlier, including the following:

- Fick CO
- Cardiac index
- Pulmonary vascular resistance (PVR)
- Pulmonary artery pulsatility index (PAPi)
- Systemic vascular resistance (SVR)
- Oxygen uptake
- Oxygen delivery
- Stroke volume
- Stroke volume index
- RAP/pulmonary arterial wedge pressure ratio
- Left ventricular stroke work index
- RV stroke work index
- Cardiac power output

Equipment

Typical PAC includes the following ports and lumens.

- The proximal injectate port is blue with a lumen in the right atrium, which is 30 cm from the catheter tip and

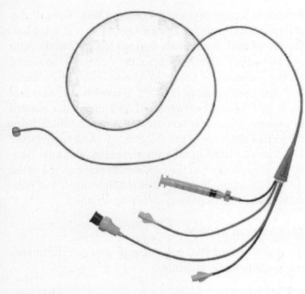

FIGURE 6-3. Pulmonary artery catheter.

helps monitor CVP/RAP and injection of cold thermo-dilution fluid.

- The distal port is yellow and is used to measure PAP and check mixed venous oxyhemoglobin saturation.
- The balloon inflation port is red and connected to a balloon syringe. It is used for balloon inflation/deflation and to check pulmonary capillary occlusive pressure.
- The pacing/infusion port is white with a lumen that terminates 31 cm from the tip of the catheter in the right atrium or RV. It is used for infusing fluids, drugs, and pacing wire.
- The thermistor connector is a red connector that includes a temperature-sensitive wire that terminates 4 cm proximal to the tip of the catheter, allowing CO determination using thermodilution.

Indications

There are several indications for PAC placement for the evaluation and management of a wide variety of cardio-vascular conditions.

- Severe cardiogenic shock (fulminant myocarditis, suspected pericardial tamponade, severe acute valvular disease, and patients requiring inotropic and vasopressor)
- Evaluation and differential diagnosis of pulmonary hypertension and to assess response to therapies
- Workup for transplantation

- Unexplained volume status in shock or suspected pseudo-sepsis
- Congenital heart disease patients who are undergoing corrective surgery
- Major cardiac surgeries (left ventricular assist device, Impella RP)

Contraindications

Relative and site-specific absolute contraindications include the following:

- Skin or soft tissue infection at the insertion site
- Endocarditis with valve vegetations on tricuspid or pulmonary valve
- RV assist device
- Severe acid-base and electrolyte disturbances that increase the risk of arrhythmias
- Insertion during cardiopulmonary bypass
- Anatomic occlusion due to a right heart mass or pulmonary thrombus
- Severe thrombocytopenia (platelet count $<50 \times 10^9/L$)
- Severe coagulopathy with INR greater than 1.5
- Agitated, uncooperative patient

Complications

Potential complications related to using PAC can occur during catheter placement, long-term maintenance, and hemodynamic data misinterpretation, and include the following:

- Looping of the catheter, knotting, or catheter misplacement
- Atrial arrhythmias, sustained ventricular arrhythmias due to irritation, right bundle branch block, and complete heart block in patients with preexisting left bundle branch block
- Pulmonary artery perforation at the moment of balloon inflation, perforation of a right atrium or ventricle, and valve rupture
- Thromboembolic events
- Catheter-related bloodstream infections, exit site infections, and endocarditis
- Venous air embolism
- Improperly leveled pressure monitors
- Migration of catheter components
- Interobserver variation in hemodynamic data interpretation
- Underinflated or overinflated balloon leading to over-estimated or underestimated PCOP, respectively

Troubleshooting

- The PAC should be zeroed and referenced before taking readings.
- The patient should preferably lie in the supine position or approximately at a 30-degree angle in a semi-recumbent position.
- Under- or overdamped waveform: Underdamping is caused by excessive tubing lengths, high-output states, or tachycardia. An overdamped waveform occurs due to air bubbles in the tubing, a kinked catheter, or when the catheter tip becomes partially occluded by the blood clot or vessel wall. These factors should be systematically addressed.
- Correct position in West's zone 3 of the lung should be ensured.
- Permanent wedge can occur, even when the balloon is deflated, due to the catheter tip being too far into the pulmonary arteriole. It should be slowly retracted as soon as possible.
- Failure to wedge due to a balloon in the larger section of the pulmonary arteriole can be fixed by slowly advancing the catheter.

Future Directions

Randomized controlled trials are required to demonstrate the effectiveness of PAC in guiding therapy in severely ill patients in the cardiac unit.

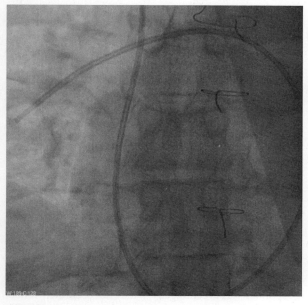

FIGURE 6-4. Fluoroscopic image showing pulmonary artery catheter.

■ VOLUME STATUS AND FLUID RESPONSIVENESS TOOLS

Invasive devices known as CVC and PAC have historically been used to assess hemodynamics, but several studies have shown that PAC fails to improve outcome in critically ill patients. Now several less invasive technologies are available for hemodynamic monitoring to assess parameters such as intravascular volume status, fluid responsiveness, CO, and tissue perfusion.

There are few commercially available noninvasive technologies for assessing fluid responsiveness and volume status. These include ultrasonography of TVC to measure diameter, lung ultrasonography for the assessment of B-lines, pulse pressure variation (PPV) measurements, and stroke volume variation (SVV).

Point-of-Care Ultrasonography of Lung

- Point-of-care ultrasonography (POCUS) of the lung is a noninvasive tool that can be used at the bedside to quickly diagnose various lung conditions, including pneumothorax, pleural effusion, pulmonary edema by visualization of B-lines, and acute respiratory distress syndrome (ARDS).
- POCUS can be performed quickly and does not require the use of ionizing radiation, making it a safer option for patients, especially for repeat imaging or for pregnant women. POCUS has proven to be a valuable tool for emergency physicians, intensivists, and pulmonologists, as it provides real-time information that can help guide patient management and improve outcomes.

■ TABLE 6-2. Various Fluid Assessment Devices

Device	Advantage	Disadvantage
Point-of-care ultrasound	Noninvasive, bedside available, quick information	Poor windows, requires skillset
Pulse pressure variation/stroke volume variation	Very effective in fluid assessment	Invasive, requires sinus rhythm and ventilated patient
Ultrasound of IVC	Noninvasive, bedside available, quick information	Not reliable in mechanically ventilated patients

- POCUS can be useful in the evaluation and management of heart failure and in the cardiac critical unit. POCUS can help healthcare providers quickly assess cardiac function, including left ventricular ejection fraction, pericardial effusion, and pulmonary edema.
- POCUS can also be used to assess the response to medical therapy in patients with heart failure. It is important to note that although POCUS is a useful tool in the evaluation and management of heart failure, it should not be used as a sole diagnostic tool.
- It is also important to note that POCUS is not a substitute for other imaging modalities and the results of POCUS should always be interpreted in conjunction with clinical findings and other imaging modalities, such as computed tomography scans and echocardiography.

Pulse Pressure Variation

- PPV is the difference between the maximum pulse pressure minus the minimum pulse pressure divided by mean pulse pressure times 100, occurring over 3 to 5 respiratory cycles.
- PPV is a valuable tool that represents an interaction between heart and lungs. The variation in pulse pressure (ie, the difference between systolic and diastolic arterial blood pressure) on an arterial line can help guide fluid management and determine fluid responsiveness in the critically ill. By monitoring changes in PPV, physicians can quickly determine the effectiveness of fluid therapy and adjust treatment as needed to optimize patient outcomes and reduce the risk of complications associated with fluid overload.
- A PPV of greater than 13% is considered predictive of fluid responsiveness, meaning the patient's stroke volume will increase with a fluid challenge. High PPV values suggest that a patient is likely to benefit from fluid administration, whereas low PPV values indicate that a patient may be volume resuscitated and that additional fluids may not be necessary.
- For appropriate measurement, the patient should be in sinus rhythm (consistent filling time) and should have sufficiently large tidal volume (at least 8 mL/kg for consistent effect of ventilator) for patients on the mechanical ventilator, passive breathing, and a good arterial waveform from arterial line.

- PPV is less reliable and should not be used in patients with cardiac arrhythmias (in atrial fibrillation, preload and pulse pressure can vary significantly beat-to-beat), spontaneous breathing (alters intrathoracic pressure unpredictably, making interpretation difficult), low tidal volume, low lung compliance, increased intra-abdominal pressure, open chest (heart/lungs interacting), RV dysfunction or conditions that affect vascular tone, and very high respiratory rate.
- One of the main disadvantages of PPV monitoring is that it requires an arterial catheter, which can be invasive and carries a risk of complications such as bleeding, infection, and thrombosis. PPV is also affected by changes in mechanical ventilation settings, which can affect the accuracy of the measurements (ie, decreased sensitivity in tidal volumes of ≤6 mL/kg). PPV has also been studied in spontaneous breathing, where it has been shown to have a diminished sensitivity but good specificity.

Stroke Volume Variation

- SVV is a measure of the variation in stroke volume, which is used to assess fluid responsiveness in mechanically ventilated patients and to guide fluid management in the critically ill.
- SVV is measured by calculating the difference between the minimum and maximum stroke volume during a respiratory cycle.
- An SVV of greater than 10% to 13% is considered predictive of fluid responsiveness, meaning that the patient's CO will increase with a fluid challenge.
- By monitoring changes in SVV, healthcare providers can quickly determine the effectiveness of fluid therapy and adjust treatment as needed to optimize patient outcomes or determine whether it may be harmful, potentially reducing the risk of complications.
- Measuring fluid responsiveness using SVV resulted in a shorter hospital stay and a reduction in mortality.
- SVV is influenced by several factors that may lead to inaccurate or misleading results. For example, changes in tidal volume, positive end-expiratory pressure (PEEP), and intrathoracic pressure can all affect SVV, regardless of a patient's fluid status.
- Additionally, in patients with low CO or significant left ventricular/RV failure, irregular heart rhythms, or spontaneous breathing, SVV may not accurately reflect fluid responsiveness.

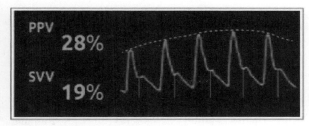

FIGURE 6-5. Stroke volume variation.

- Finally, the use of SVV may require specialized equipment and expertise, which may not be readily available in all healthcare settings.
- It is important to note that SVV and PPV are not perfect predictors of fluid responsiveness, and other factors, such as the presence of intrinsic PEEP, must be taken into consideration.
- Additionally, SVV and PPV should not be used as a sole diagnostic tool, and its results should always be interpreted in conjunction with clinical findings and other monitoring parameters.

Oximetric Waveform Variation

- Oximetric waveform variation, also known as pulse oximetry variation, is a measure of the variation (difference between the minimum and maximum amplitude of the pulse oximetry waveform) from a plethysmograph during a respiratory cycle.
- Pulse oximetry is a noninvasive technique used to monitor a patient's oxygen saturation, the amount of oxygen in the blood. A large oximetric waveform variation can indicate fluid responsiveness, meaning that the patient's stroke volume will increase with a fluid challenge.
- Oximetric waveform variation can be used to help guide fluid management in critically ill patients, particularly in those who are mechanically ventilated.
- By monitoring the changes in the oximetry waveform, clinicians can make informed decisions about fluid management, such as whether to administer fluids or adjust ventilation settings.

Ultrasonography of Thoracic Vena Cava

Ultrasonography of the TVC can be used to estimate a patient's intravascular volume status, and the size and collapsibility of the TVC can provide information about the volume status of the circulatory system.

By measuring the diameter of the inferior vena cava (IVC), healthcare providers can estimate the volume of blood returning to the heart and, by extension, the CO.

To perform a TVC ultrasound, a trained ultrasonographer will apply a transducer to the patient's neck or chest and visualize the TVC in real time.

The diameter of the TVC will be measured at end-expiration and end-inspiration, and the variation in diameter will be used to estimate CO. A distended IVC with little collapsibility is suggestive of hypervolemia, whereas a collapsed IVC is indicative of hypovolemia.

While assessment of the IVC can be a useful tool for estimating a patient's intravascular volume status, there are some potential pitfalls to be aware of.

- First, the IVC is influenced by factors other than volume status, such as changes in intrathoracic pressure, cardiac function, and RAP. These factors can affect the size and collapsibility of the IVC, even in the absence of significant changes in volume status.
- Second, there is a lack of standardized criteria for IVC assessment, with different studies using different measurement techniques and cutoff values. This can lead to variability in the interpretation of IVC findings, making it challenging to use this tool to guide clinical decision-making.

Overall, although IVC assessment can be a useful adjunct to other methods of volume assessment, it should not be used in isolation and requires careful interpretation in the context of the individual patient's clinical situation.

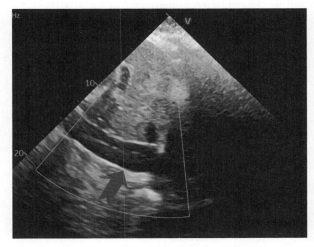

FIGURE 6-6. Dilated IVC showing elevated filling pressures.

> ■ **TABLE 6-3. Devices for Cardiac Output Monitoring**
>
> - Lithium dilution–based devices
> - Thermodilution-based devices
> - Thoracic electrical bioreactance or bioimpedance
> - Aortic Doppler
> - Focused cardiac ultrasound

Cardiac Output Measurement

CO is the amount of blood pumped by the heart per minute. Normal output is 5 to 6 L/min. In patients with hemodynamic instability, CO is a useful parameter to guide intravascular volume and etiology of illness.

Several commercially available noninvasive technologies have been developed to calculate CO. These devices assess CO based on the arterial pulse waveform, thoracic electrical bioimpedance, and bioreactance. Arterial waveform-based devices include lithium dilution–based devices and thermodilution-based devices. CO may be calculated by transesophagus or transcutaneous aortic Doppler and point-of-care echocardiography by determining the velocity-time integral at the level of the left ventricular outflow tract.

Lithium Dilution–Based Devices

Lithium dilution CO (LiDCO) is a hemodynamic monitoring system that uses the lithium dilution method to measure CO and other hemodynamic parameters.

Mechanism of Action In the LiDCO system, a small amount of lithium chloride is injected into a central vein, and its concentration is measured in the arterial blood over time using a specialized LiDCO monitor. The dilution of the lithium in the blood reflects the CO, as the amount of blood pumped by the heart dilutes the lithium and decreases its concentration in the blood. The LiDCO monitor also uses a proprietary algorithm to calculate other hemodynamic parameters, such as stroke volume, SVV, and systemic vascular resistance, based on the lithium dilution data and other patient-specific information entered into the system.

Indications The LiDCO system can be used in a variety of clinical settings, including critical care, anesthesia, and perioperative care. It is designed to provide continuous and accurate hemodynamic monitoring to guide clinical decision-making and optimize patient outcomes.

However, like any hemodynamic monitoring system, the LiDCO system has its limitations and should be used in conjunction with other clinical and laboratory data to make informed patient management decisions. Overreliance on the LiDCO system without considering other factors may lead to incorrect or inappropriate patient management decisions.

Complications Although LiDCO is a useful tool for hemodynamic monitoring, there are some potential pitfalls to be aware of.

- First, the accuracy of the LiDCO system can be affected by a number of factors, including changes in vascular resistance or pulmonary blood flow, as well as technical factors such as accurate measurement of the lithium concentration and ensuring complete mixing of the lithium in the blood.
- Second, the LiDCO system is a complex and relatively expensive technology and requires specialized training to operate and interpret the data. As such, it may not be readily available or feasible to use in all clinical settings.

Troubleshooting Troubleshooting LiDCO can involve several steps to identify and resolve issues with the system. Here are some troubleshooting tips:

- Ensure proper setup: Check that the LiDCO monitor is correctly set up and calibrated, with the appropriate patient data entered into the system. Make sure that the lithium chloride solution is prepared and injected according to the manufacturer's instructions.
- Check for technical issues: If the LiDCO system is not providing accurate readings, check for technical issues such as a faulty monitor or probe, inadequate mixing of the lithium in the blood, or interference from other equipment.
- Assess patient factors: Inaccurate readings can also be caused by patient-related factors, such as changes in vascular resistance or pulmonary blood flow, or by certain cardiac or pulmonary conditions. Assess the patient's clinical status and consider whether other factors may be affecting the accuracy of the LiDCO measurements.
- Verify with other methods: If you suspect that the LiDCO measurements are inaccurate, verify them with other methods such as thermodilution or Doppler ultrasound. This can help identify any discrepancies and ensure that accurate measurements are being obtained.
- Consult technical support: If troubleshooting efforts are unsuccessful, contact the LiDCO technical support team for assistance with resolving the issue.

Overall, troubleshooting LiDCO involves a systematic approach to identify and resolve any issues with the system, ensuring that accurate hemodynamic measurements are obtained to guide clinical decision-making.

Thermodilution-Based Devices

Thermodilution-based devices are a type of technology used to measure CO in critically ill patients.

Mechanism of Action

- These devices work by introducing a small amount of cold saline into the bloodstream and measuring the change in temperature of the saline as it passes through the heart. The change in temperature is used to calculate CO.
- To perform a thermodilution measurement, a small catheter is inserted into a peripheral vein, and a bolus of cold saline is injected into the bloodstream.
- The temperature change of the saline is then measured as it passes through the heart and is used to calculate CO.

Indications and Contraindications

- Thermodilution-based devices are a useful tool in the management of critically ill patients, as they can quickly provide information about CO, which is a key factor in determining fluid responsiveness and guiding fluid management.
- Additionally, these devices are relatively noninvasive, allowing for real-time monitoring of CO without the need for more invasive procedures.

Complications and Troubleshooting

- It is important to note that thermodilution-based devices should not be used as a sole diagnostic tool, and their results should always be interpreted in conjunction with clinical findings and other monitoring parameters.
- Additionally, the accuracy of thermodilution-based devices can be affected by a variety of factors, including patient positioning and the presence of intrinsic PEEP.

Thoracic Electrical Bioreactance or Bioimpedance

Thoracic electrical bioimpedance (TEB) is a noninvasive method of measuring CO in critically ill patients. TEB uses electrical currents to estimate the volume of blood in the thorax and, by extension, the CO.

TEB devices consist of 2 electrodes, one placed on the right shoulder and the other on the left ankle. A small electrical current is passed between the electrodes, and the resistance of the current is measured. The resistance is proportional to the volume of blood in the thorax and can be used to calculate CO.

TEB is a useful tool in the management of critically ill patients, as it can quickly provide information about CO, which is a key factor in determining fluid responsiveness and guiding fluid management.

Additionally, TEB is noninvasive and can be performed at the bedside, allowing for real-time monitoring of CO without the need for more invasive procedures. It is important to note that TEB should not be used as a sole diagnostic tool, and its results should always be interpreted in conjunction with clinical findings and other monitoring parameters. Additionally, the accuracy of TEB can be affected by a variety of factors, including patient positioning and the presence of intrinsic PEEP.

Aortic Doppler

Aortic Doppler ultrasound is a method of measuring CO by evaluating blood flow in the aorta.

Mechanism of Action The Doppler ultrasound technique uses high-frequency sound waves to measure the velocity of blood flow in the aorta. The velocity of blood flow is proportional to the stroke volume, which is the volume of blood pumped out of the heart with each beat. By multiplying the stroke volume by the heart rate, the CO can be calculated.

Aortic Doppler ultrasound is performed using a transducer that is placed on the chest over the aortic arch. The ultrasound beam is directed toward the aorta, and the velocity of blood flow is measured as it passes through the transducer. The resulting Doppler waveform is used to calculate the stroke volume and, ultimately, the CO.

Indications and Contraindications Aortic Doppler ultrasound is a useful tool in the management of critically ill patients, as it can quickly provide information about CO, which is a key factor in determining fluid responsiveness and guiding fluid management. Additionally, Doppler ultrasound is noninvasive and can be performed at the bedside, allowing for real-time monitoring of CO without the need for more invasive procedures.

Complications and Troubleshooting It is important to note that aortic Doppler ultrasound should not be used as a sole diagnostic tool, and its results should always be interpreted in conjunction with clinical findings and other monitoring parameters.

Additionally, the accuracy of aortic Doppler ultrasound can be affected by a variety of factors, including patient positioning and the presence of intrinsic PEEP.

Focused Cardiac Ultrasound

Focused cardiac ultrasound (FCU) refers to the use of bedside ultrasound technology to obtain real-time images of the heart. This method of imaging is becoming increasingly popular in the management of critically ill patients, as it can provide important information about the function of the heart and surrounding structures, including the valves, pericardium, and great vessels.

Mechanism of Action FCU can be performed using a handheld ultrasound device that is portable and easy to use. This allows for the acquisition of images at the bedside, without the need for transporting the patient to a radiology suite. This is particularly beneficial in critically ill patients, as it allows for real-time monitoring of cardiac function and the ability to respond quickly to changes in the patient's condition.

Indications and Contraindications The images obtained using FCU can provide information about a variety of cardiac parameters, including the size and shape of the chambers, the motion of the walls, the blood flow in the vessels, and the function of the valves. This information can be used to diagnose and monitor conditions such as heart failure, valvular disease, and cardiac tamponade.

Complications and Troubleshooting It is important to note that FCU should not be used as a sole diagnostic tool, and its results should always be interpreted in conjunction with clinical findings and other monitoring parameters.

■ TISSUE PERFUSION

Measurement of Microcirculatory Blood Flow

Shock-induced microcirculatory dysfunction is a condition that occurs when blood flow to the small blood vessels, known as the microcirculation, is impaired in response to a state of shock. This can result in poor perfusion of tissues and organs, leading to cellular hypoxia and metabolic imbalances that can contribute to the development of organ dysfunction.

Shock can be caused by a variety of conditions, including sepsis, cardiogenic shock, hypovolemic shock, and obstructive shock. In each of these conditions, the body's

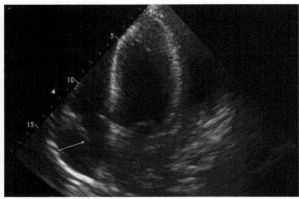

A

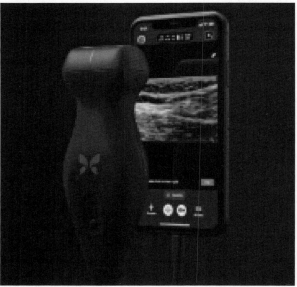

B

FIGURE 6-7. Focused cardiac ultrasound image (**A**) and device (**B**).

response to the shock state can result in the development of microcirculatory dysfunction, which can further exacerbate the severity of the shock state.

Microcirculatory dysfunction is associated with an increased risk of morbidity and mortality in patients with shock. It is therefore important to assess the microcirculation in these patients and to monitor it over time in order to identify any changes in perfusion and to guide therapeutic interventions aimed at improving microcirculatory blood flow.

There are various techniques that can be used to assess microcirculatory blood flow, including laser speckle contrast imaging, near-infrared spectroscopy, and the assessment of sublingual capillary refill time. Each of these techniques has its own advantages and limitations, and it is important to choose the most appropriate method based on the patient's specific needs and clinical situation.

In conclusion, shock-induced microcirculatory dysfunction is a common and serious complication of shock, and early recognition and management are essential in order to improve patient outcomes.

Capillary Refill Versus Lactate

Capillary refill time (CRT) and lactate levels are 2 commonly used markers in the evaluation and management of shock. Both of these measures can provide important information about the state of perfusion in critically ill patients and can help guide therapeutic decisions.

CRT refers to the time it takes for color to return to the nail bed after it has been compressed and released. A prolonged CRT is a sign of decreased perfusion and can indicate the presence of shock or the development of microcirculatory dysfunction. CRT is a simple and noninvasive measure that can be performed at the bedside, making it an attractive option for monitoring perfusion in critically ill patients.

Lactate levels, on the other hand, are a measure of anaerobic metabolism and can provide information about the severity of hypoperfusion in critically ill patients. Elevated lactate levels are a sign of poor tissue perfusion and are associated with an increased risk of morbidity and mortality in patients with shock. Lactate levels can be measured using a blood sample, making it a more invasive measure than CRT.

In conclusion, both CRT and lactate levels are important markers in the evaluation and management of shock. CRT is a simple and noninvasive measure that can provide valuable information about perfusion, while lactate levels provide a more quantitative measure of the severity of hypoperfusion. The choice of which measure to use will depend on the clinical situation and the needs of the patient.

Measurement of Tissue Oxygen Saturation

Measurement of tissue oxygen saturation (StO_2) is a useful tool in the evaluation and management of shock. StO_2 refers to the oxygen saturation of the microcirculation, which is the small blood vessels that supply oxygen and nutrients to tissues and organs.

In patients with shock, low StO_2 levels are associated with an increased risk of morbidity and mortality. Early recognition of low StO_2 levels and initiation of appropriate therapeutic interventions can help to improve perfusion and reduce the risk of organ dysfunction in these patients. StO_2 can be assessed using near-infrared spectroscopy (NIRS).

Near-Infrared Spectroscopy

Measurement of StO_2 using NIRS is a valuable tool in the evaluation and management of shock. It provides real-time, continuous, and noninvasive information about tissue perfusion that can be used to guide therapeutic decisions and improve patient outcomes.

Mechanism of Action StO_2 can be measured using NIRS, which involves the use of light to assess the oxygen saturation of tissues. NIRS works by shining light of different wavelengths into the tissue and measuring the amount of light that is absorbed and scattered. NIRS measures the relative amounts of oxygenated and deoxygenated hemoglobin in tissues, and from this information, it calculates the StO_2. The normal range is 60% to 75%.

Indications and Contraindications The technique is safe and noninvasive and can be performed at the bedside, making it an attractive option for monitoring tissue perfusion in critically ill patients.

NIRS has been used in a variety of clinical settings, including critical care, surgery, and sports medicine. In critical care, NIRS is used to monitor tissue perfusion

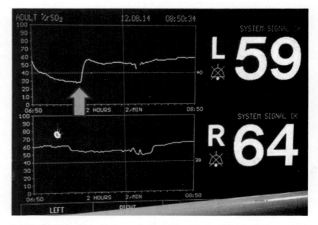

FIGURE 6-8. Near-infrared spectroscopy of lower extremity in extracorporeal membrane oxygenation patient.

in patients with shock, sepsis, and other conditions that can lead to microcirculatory dysfunction and cellular hypoxia.

By providing real-time, continuous, and noninvasive information about tissue perfusion, NIRS can be used to guide therapeutic decisions and improve patient outcomes.

Complications and Troubleshooting The results should always be interpreted in conjunction with clinical findings and other monitoring parameters.

■ MANAGEMENT OF FLUID OVERLOAD STATUS AND FLUID REMOVAL DEVICES

Following are the methods for removing extra fluid inside the body when diuretic therapy fails to work.

Aquapheresis

Heart failure is a condition in which the heart is unable to pump blood effectively, leading to fluid buildup in the body. This fluid buildup, known as edema, can cause symptoms such as shortness of breath, fatigue, and swelling in the legs, ankles, and feet. Aquapheresis can be used to quickly and effectively remove this excess fluid, reducing symptoms and improving quality of life.

Mechanism of Action

The aquapheresis procedure involves using a dialysis-like machine to remove fluid from the bloodstream. The blood is passed through a membrane that filters out excess fluid, which is then discarded. The cleaned blood is then returned to the body.

In the case of heart failure, aquapheresis is used to help alleviate fluid overload and improve symptoms.

Equipment
- Aquadex flow pump
- Single use circuit
- Heparin saline
- 6-F, dual-lumen, extended-length peripheral catheter

Indications and Contraindications

Aquapheresis is indicated for patients with heart failure who have refractory fluid overload and severe symptoms such as shortness of breath, fatigue, and impaired quality of life. The procedure should only be performed under the supervision of a healthcare provider with experience in aquapheresis and in a setting equipped to manage potential complications.

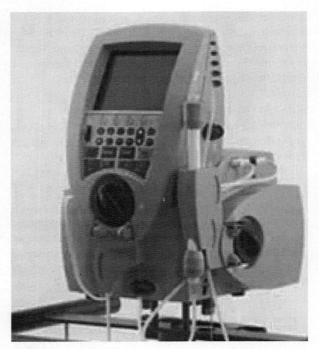

FIGURE 6-9. Aquapheresis setup. (See color insert.)

Aquapheresis is not suitable for everyone, and there are several contraindications to the procedure in heart failure patients. Some of the most common contraindications include:

- Active bleeding: Aquapheresis can increase the risk of bleeding and is not recommended in patients with active bleeding.
- Low blood pressure: The procedure can lower blood pressure and is not recommended in patients with low blood pressure.
- Severe anemia: Aquapheresis can lead to a decrease in red blood cell count and is not recommended in patients with severe anemia.
- Severe electrolyte imbalances: The procedure can disrupt electrolyte balance and is not recommended in patients with severe electrolyte imbalances.
- Unstable heart condition: Aquapheresis can be physically stressful and is not recommended in patients with an unstable heart condition.
- Recent surgery: The procedure can increase the risk of bleeding and is not recommended in patients who have recently undergone surgery.
- Pregnancy: Aquapheresis is not recommended in pregnant women due to the potential for harm to the fetus.

Complications and Troubleshooting

- There is a risk for access-related issues such as vascular injury, bleeding, pneumothorax, and venous thrombosis and risk of heparin-induced thrombocytopenia.
- Priming the port is required when the machine gives an alert; make sure to remove any air.
- When the machine shows withdrawing difficulty or withdrawal line occlusion, make sure to check the position of catheter tip, check for clots in the circuit, remove kinks in tubing, verify clamps are open, and avoid excessive motion.

Future Directions

Efforts are ongoing to improve the circuit complexity and ease of use and troubleshoot the system, which will make its use more common in routine settings.

Continuous Venovenous Hemofiltration

Continuous venovenous hemofiltration (CVVH) is typically performed in an intensive care unit and is typically used as a last resort for critically ill patients who are unable to maintain adequate blood flow and oxygenation despite medical treatment. The procedure is often used in combination with other treatments, such as medications and mechanical ventilation, to support the patient's recovery.

Mechanism of Action

CVVH is similar to continuous renal replacement therapy, but it is designed to provide more comprehensive filtration of the blood using a semi-permeable membrane in a slow fashion. It works on the principle of diffusion and convection.

Equipment and Technique

- In CVVH, a catheter is inserted into a large vein, typically the internal jugular or femoral vein. Blood is then pumped from the vein through a filter, where waste products, excess fluid, and toxins are removed. The cleaned blood is then returned to the patient's bloodstream.
- Anticoagulation is utilized by using heparin to avoid microthrombi in the circuit. Citrate anticoagulation can be used with caution regarding calcium depletion.
- All the alarms should be addressed before initiation of therapy.
- Drug dosing should be carefully sought during CVVH therapy, and doses should be adjusted for clinical effects, avoiding toxicity.

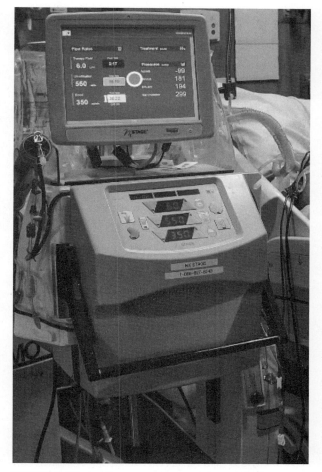

FIGURE 6-10. Continuous venovenous hemofiltration setup. (See color insert.)

Indications and Contraindications

CVVH is used to treat a variety of conditions, including acute heart failure, cardiac arrest, sepsis, and other life-threatening conditions that result in organ failure. The procedure can help to remove fluid, waste products, and toxins from the bloodstream, improving organ function and reducing the risk of organ failure.

CVVH is indicated in cardiac critical care units for patients with life-threatening conditions that result in organ failure and require extensive filtration of the blood. CVVH is used to treat conditions such as the following:

- Acute heart failure: CVVH can help remove excess fluid from the bloodstream in patients with heart failure, reducing the workload on the heart and improving CO.

- Cardiac arrest: CVVH can help remove toxins and waste products from the bloodstream in patients who have suffered a cardiac arrest, improving organ function and reducing the risk of organ failure.
- Severe sepsis: CVVH can help remove waste products and toxins from the bloodstream in patients with severe sepsis, reducing the risk of organ failure and improving the patient's chances of recovery.
- Other life-threatening conditions: CVVH can be used to treat other conditions, such as liver failure, kidney failure, and multiple organ failure, in which the patient's organs are unable to function properly.

Despite its potential benefits, there are certain contraindications for CVVH that must be considered before the procedure is performed. Some of these contraindications include the following:

- Coagulopathy: Patients with a history of bleeding disorders or who are taking anticoagulants may not be suitable candidates for CVVH, as the procedure may increase the risk of bleeding.
- Hemodynamic instability: CVVH may not be suitable for patients who are experiencing severe hemodynamic instability, as the procedure may cause further instability.
- Arteriovenous fistulas: Patients with a history of arteriovenous fistulas or other vascular access-related complications may not be suitable candidates for CVVH, as the procedure may increase the risk of these complications.
- Severe electrolyte imbalances: Patients with severe electrolyte imbalances, such as low potassium levels, may not be suitable candidates for CVVH, as the procedure may worsen these imbalances.
- Hypotension: Patients with severe hypotension may not be suitable candidates for CVVH, as the procedure may worsen this condition.

It is important to note that these are general contraindications and the suitability of CVVH for a particular patient will depend on a number of factors, including the patient's overall health, medical history, and the severity of their condition. A thorough evaluation by a healthcare provider is necessary before the procedure is performed.

Complications
- Local bleeding and vascular access injury that may need monitoring of hemoglobin.
- Hypothermia due to fluid shift. Warmer may be applied in the circuit.

- Electrolyte imbalance. Every 6 to 8 hours, pH and electrolyte check required in first 24 hours.
- Risk of infection that requires monitoring of fever and local swelling.

Troubleshooting
- Access pressure is usually negative, and excessive negative pressure should warrant assessment of catheter position, kinks in tubing, patient position, and aspiration with manual flushing.
- Changes in return circuit positive pressure require similar checks as described earlier.
- Filter pressure alarm signifies clot in the filter requiring change of filter.
- The sensor alarm can detect myoglobin in the circuit requiring further assessment.
- The bubble detector will stop the pump if air is detected requiring re-priming and de-airing the system.

Future Directions
Ethical concerns regarding withdrawal of therapy are an ongoing area of discussion in crucially ill patients. Strategies of anticoagulation also require uniformity across the clinical practice.

SUGGESTED READINGS

Marik PE. Techniques for assessment of intravascular volume in critically ill patients. *J Intensive Care Med.* 2009;24(5):329-337.

Tolwani A. Continuous renal-replacement therapy for acute kidney injury. *N Engl J Med.* 2012;367(26):2505-2514.

Abbreviations

CO: Cardiac output
CRT: Capillary refill time
CVC: Central venous catheter
CVP: Central venous pressure
CVVH: Continuous venovenous hemofiltration
FCU: Focused cardiac ultrasound
INR: International normalized ratio
IVC: Inferior vena cava
LiDCO: Lithium dilution cardiac output
mPAP: Mean pulmonary artery pressure
NIRS: Near-infrared spectroscopy
PAC: Pulmonary artery catheter
PAH: Pulmonary arterial hypertension
PAP: Pulmonary arterial pressure
PCOP: Pulmonary capillary occlusive pressure

PEEP: Positive end expiratory pressure
POCUS: Point-of-care ultrasonography
PPV: Pulse pressure variation
PVR: Pulmonary vascular resistance
RAP: Right atrial pressure
RHC: Right heart catheterization

RV: Right ventricle
StO_2: Tissue oxygen saturation
SVV: Stroke volume variation
TEB: Thoracic electrical bioimpedance
TVC: Thoracic vena cava

Devices for Management of Acute Pulmonary Embolism

• *Vibha Hayagreev, MD; Iqra Bhatti, MD; Preeti Jadhav, MD; Charbel Ishak, MD; Timothy J. Vittorio, MD; Sneha Khannal, MD*

■ CASE PRESENTATION

A 65-year-old woman presents to the emergency department with acute onset of dyspnea, chest pain, and palpitations. Comorbidities include coronary artery disease, hypertension, and uterine cancer. The patient currently takes metoprolol, lisinopril, and aspirin. On examination, she is tachycardic, tachypneic, and hypoxic.

Blood pressure is 122/84 mmHg. Electrocardiogram shows sinus tachycardia. Chest X-ray shows no acute cardiopulmonary pathology. Computed tomography for pulmonary embolism shows acute pulmonary embolism.

The patient is admitted to intensive care unit for further management while being referred to interventionist for percutaneous treatment and evaluation for catheter-directed thrombolysis.

■ KEY POINTS

- Acute pulmonary embolism is a well-known medical condition in hospital that can result in adverse clinical outcomes. Cardiac patients are at risk of this complication due to their comorbid condition.
- In addition to anticoagulation, mechanical thrombectomy devices have been introduced to analyze the benefit of clot retrieval on overall cardiopulmonary function.
- Prophylaxis should be implemented to prevent thromboembolic events during or after hospitalization.

■ INTRODUCTION

Pulmonary embolism (PE) is one of the most common causes of death worldwide. PEs can get lodged in the pulmonary trunk, main pulmonary artery, or segmental or subsegmental branches.

Based on the size and location of the thrombi, hemodynamic changes such as increased right heart pressures, increased pulmonary artery pressures, and decreased diffusing capacity of the lungs for carbon monoxide are seen. Saddle emboli are known to have the most severe consequences due to their size and anatomic location, which can sequentially block the right and left pulmonary arteries, leading to severe obstruction of right heart outflow tract.

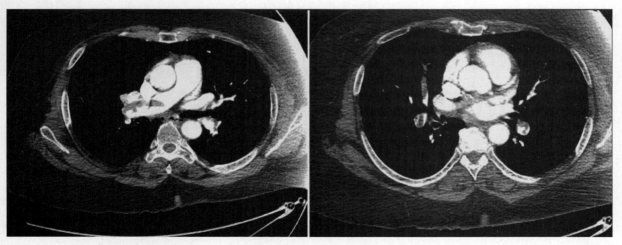

FIGURE 7-1. Saddle embolisms are seen within the distal aspect of the right main pulmonary artery extending into the right and left segmental arteries.

Catheter-directed thrombolysis (CDT) is one of the newest approaches for PE, and it can be more efficacious than anticoagulation alone. In addition, CDT appears to be safer than systemic thrombolysis, and procedure-related complications are very rare.

■ CATHETER-DIRECTED THROMBOLYSIS

Review of Literature

- Studies show that right-sided pressures are similar at 3 months for patients treated with CDT or with anticoagulation alone.
- Given the minimal rate of procedure-related complications, CDT appears to have lower bleeding risk than systemic thrombolysis for the treatment of intermediate-risk PE.
- However, there may be increased major bleeding compared with anticoagulation alone. CDT is associated with a low mortality rate (up to 4%), but the mortality rate for patients treated with anticoagulation alone is similar.
- CDT not only improves clinical outcomes in patients with acute PE but also minimizes the risk of major bleeding.
- Patients with acute massive and submassive PE can be managed with ultrasound-guided, catheter-directed, low-dose fibrinolysis because it decreases right ventricular (RV) dilation, pulmonary hypertension, and thrombus burden and minimizes intracranial hemorrhage.

Mechanism of Action

- CDT is a percutaneous procedure in which a thrombolytic is infused via a vein directly to the clot to decrease the size and burden of the clot. The thrombolytic acts on the fibrin product and causes clot resolution.
- Ultrasound-assisted thrombolytic delivery can also be achieved using the Ekosonic endovascular catheter (Boston Scientific).

Equipment

- Introducer kit and access kit
- EKOS catheter or pigtail catheter
- Closure devices

Indications

CDT is a class 2C recommendation by the American College of Chest Physicians for the management of acute PE in the following patient groups: patients with hypotension and who have contraindications to thrombolysis; patients with failed thrombolysis; and patients with shock that is likely to cause death before systemic thrombolysis can take effect (eg, within hours) and if appropriate expertise and resources are available. This includes massive and intermediate-high submassive risk groups. It can also be used in patients with deep vein thrombosis (DVT) to reduce clot burden and reduces the risk of post-DVT syndrome.

Contraindications

- Prior ischemic stroke, cerebral bleed, or cerebral mass
- Vascular deformation

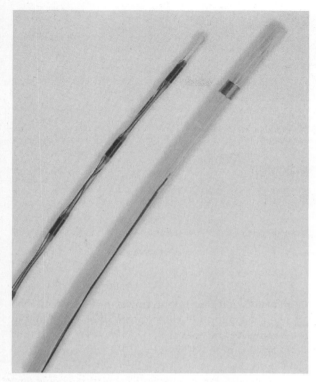

FIGURE 7-2. EKOS catheter used for CDT. (See color insert.)

- Recent ulcer in the gastrointestinal tract
- Recent brain/spine surgery
- Major abdominal or pelvic surgery
- Any source of active bleeding

Procedure

Vascular access is obtained via femoral or jugular approach using a 7- to 8-F sheath. Introducer needle is inserted into the desired venous vasculature through which a hydrophilic guidewire is threaded in. The guidewire is then directed into the pulmonary system adjacent to the thrombus via the right heart.

The infusion catheter is passed over the guidewire and across the treatment site under fluoroscopic guidance. The radiopaque marker bands at each end of the catheter enhance the catheter placement. The guidewire is removed once position is confirmed.

The interventionist inserts the ultrasonic core into the catheter until the fittings lock into place, after which thrombolytic is administered. The thrombolytic is released through side holes, while saline is administered through the distal tip of the catheter.

Dispersion of thrombolytic is enhanced by ultrasonic wave activation. Thrombolytics are typically administered for up to 18 hours along with systemic heparin; however, the duration varies based on thrombus burden and hemodynamics.

Repeat computed tomography angiography is performed to assess improvement in thrombus burden.

Once deemed complete, the ultrasonic core is removed, and the guidewire is replaced inside the catheter. The catheter is then removed, leaving the guidewire in, which is ultimately replaced, and a compression device is placed over the access site.

Complications

- Hemorrhagic stroke (one of the most common and most feared complications)
- Vascular access–related complications such as hematoma, pulmonary hemorrhage, and retroperitoneal hemorrhage
- Perforation or dissection of the pulmonary artery, arrhythmias, right-sided valvular regurgitation, pericardial tamponade, and contrast-induced nephropathy

Troubleshooting

- Heparin or systemic anticoagulation is sometimes continued after the procedure for 24 to 48 hours to prevent re-thrombosis depending on the status of the clot.
- Patient should be monitored for signs of bleeding and intracranial bleeding.
- Complete blood count (CBC) and coagulation studies should be watched carefully.
- Patient should be monitored for contrast-induced nephropathy.

Future Directions

Further trials are needed to determine if catheter-directed therapy reduces mortality compared with anticoagulation alone.

■ PERCUTANEOUS MECHANICAL THROMBECTOMY FOR TREATMENT OF ACUTE PULMONARY EMBOLISM

Introduction

Acute PE can present with a wide spectrum of manifestations, as shown in Figure 7-3.

Depending on the size and location, PE can cause significant changes in hemodynamics, and if the right heart system is involved, echocardiogram will show flattening

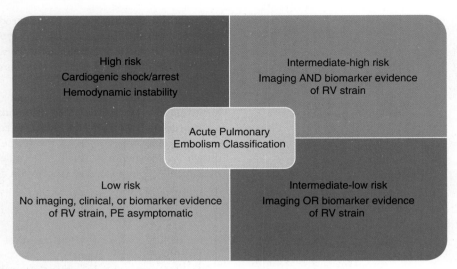

FIGURE 7-3. Acute PE classification.

of the intraventricular septum, which can be a crucial finding for appropriate and emergent intervention.

Acute PE can be treated via minimally invasive procedures such as CDT, percutaneous embolectomy, ultrasound-assisted thrombolysis, percutaneous mechanical thrombus fragmentation, and surgical embolectomy. Percutaneous mechanical thrombectomy is a novel technique designed to use in PE patients who have contraindications for thrombolysis or anticoagulation.

Mechanism of Action

A catheter is used to mechanically remove the clot using high velocity either by creating suction vacuum or physically disrupting the clot using unsheathed disks.

Indications and Contraindications

Mechanical thrombectomy is used in intermediate- to high-risk PE patients who have contraindications for systemic anticoagulation.

It is a safe and minimally invasive treatment option for acute intermediate- to high-risk PE and is associated with

immediate significant improvement in the RV/left ventricular (LV) ratio and rapid normalization of pulmonary artery pressure and SpO_2.

It can also be used in cases of PE with concomitant clots in transit.

Patients who can receive anticoagulation should not undergo this treatment in preference to avoid anticoagulation. Cardiac arrest patients with prolonged cardiopulmonary resuscitation time should be carefully selected for this procedure.

Equipment

There are 2 types of devices available:

- FlowTriever (Inari Medical, Irvine, CA) catheter
- Penumbra Indigo (Penumbra, Alameda, CA) catheter

Procedure

The FlowTriever catheter is a large-bore device that mechanically engages the thrombus in the pulmonary arteries. Once it is engaged into the vessel, 3

■ TABLE 7-1. Characteristics of Mechanical Thrombectomy Devices			
Catheter	Sheath Size	Characteristic	Benefits
FlowTriever	20 F	Nitinol disks disrupt the clot	No tissue plasminogen activator required Improves RV/LV ratio
Penumbra	4-8 F	High-velocity suction aspiration	Small caliber Less risk of bleeding

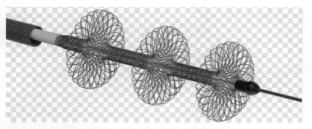

FIGURE 7-4. Inari FlowTriever catheter. (See color insert.)

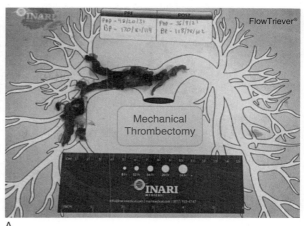

self-expanding nitinol disks are deployed. These disks are then retracted back into the catheter with the entrapped thrombus. While retracting back, synchronous aspiration is performed through the catheter to ensure the removal of thrombus en bloc from the pulmonary arteries without the use of adjunctive thrombolytics.

Complications

- Vascular access–related complications such as hematoma, pulmonary hemorrhage, and retroperitoneal hemorrhage
- Perforation or dissection of the pulmonary artery, arrhythmias, right-sided valvular regurgitation, pericardial tamponade, and contrast-induced nephropathy

Troubleshooting

- Patient should be monitored for signs of bleeding, especially intracranial bleeding.
- CBC and coagulation studies should be watched carefully.
- Patient should be monitored for contrast-induced nephropathy.

Future Directions

A head-to-head randomized trial needs to be conducted on the mechanical thrombectomy device to compare its effectiveness and long-term mortality benefits to anticoagulants and systemic thrombolytic therapy.

■ INFERIOR VENA CAVA FILTERS

Introduction

Most PEs are generated through DVTs in the lower extremities. It is generally believed that, to avoid PE, one should avoid embolization of DVT from the legs. Although it remains controversial, inferior vena cava (IVC) filters are used to prevent clot propagation.

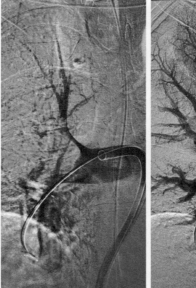
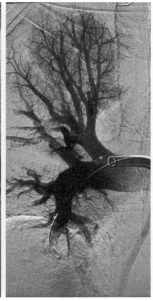

FIGURE 7-5. A, B. Clot retrieved from Inari catheter.

Mechanism of Action

An IVC filter is a metallic mesh that is inserted in the IVC and prevents clot transition to the lungs and heart.

Equipment

There are 2 types of IVC filters:

- Retrievable: Can be removed once the indication has been improved.
- Permanent: Used if there are long-term contraindications for anticoagulation.

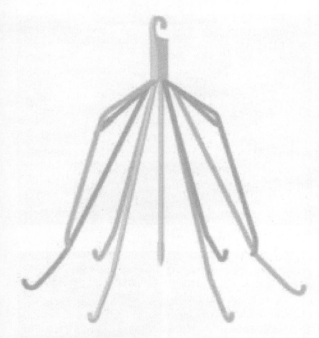

FIGURE 7-6. IVC filter.

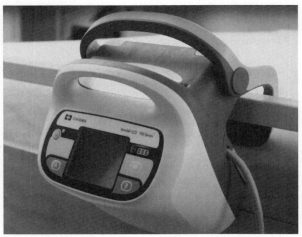

A

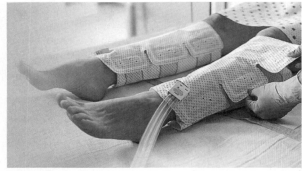

B

FIGURE 7-7. A, B. Pneumatic compression device. (See color insert.)

Indications and Contraindications

General indications include the following:

- Acute proximal DVT or PE with contraindication for anticoagulation
- Patients with massive PE with poor cardiopulmonary reserves
- Patient with recurrent DVT with failed anticoagulation

Contraindications include coagulopathy, active infection, IVC thrombosis, cancer extending to IVC, or inability to access IVC.

Complications and Troubleshooting

- An IVC filter can be a nidus for thrombus formation, vasculature injury/perforation, bowel or aorta injury, or migration into heart or lungs.
- Access site bleeding can occur after the procedure and should be monitored.
- Retrievable filters can be removed in 6 months once the condition is improved.
- X-ray or advanced imaging is required if IVC migration is suspected.

Future Directions

Advanced retrievable filters are being studied to improve the overall design to avoid thrombus formation and for utilization in primary prevention in certain situations.

■ DEEP VEIN THROMBOSIS AND PULMONARY EMBOLISM PREVENTION DEVICES

Compression Stockings and Devices

In cardiac critical care, compression stockings and devices are used to help prevent DVT and other complications related to blood clots. DVT is a serious condition that occurs when a blood clot forms in the deep veins of the legs. This can be a complication in critically ill patients, especially those who have been immobile for long periods, as well as in patients who have had surgery or a stroke, heart failure, or cancer.

Mechanism of Action

Compression stockings and devices work by applying graduated compression to the legs, which helps to improve blood flow and reduce the risk of blood clots. The reduction is most significant at the ankle and gradually decreases up the leg. This helps to push blood up the legs and toward the heart.

Indications and Contraindications

Compression stockings are typically worn during the day and can be made of materials such as nylon or elastic. They come in different sizes and compression levels and should be fitted by a healthcare professional. They can be used for bed-bound patients or postoperative patients who have limited mobility.

Compression devices, such as pneumatic and intermittent pneumatic compression, pump air into cuffs wrapped around the legs and the feet. These devices can be used for long-term prophylaxis and to treat established DVT.

It is worth noting that compression stockings and devices are not suitable for everyone, and it is essential for healthcare professionals to evaluate each patient individually to assess if it is appropriate for the patient and to monitor for any complications that may occur as a result of use, such as skin damage or impaired circulation.

In acute DVT, it is thought that compression devices should not be placed because they may dislodge the DVT. Use of compression devices on an active skin infection and open wound may cause further worsening, so they should be used carefully.

Complications and Troubleshooting

Compression devices are associated with risk of fall, skin ulceration, and limited mobility.

As per multisociety guidelines, pharmacologic prophylaxis is preferred over mechanical prophylaxis for DVT prophylaxis in critically ill patients.

Future Directions

More data are required regarding use of mechanical devices in low-risk patients and the preferred choice of device (pneumatic vs gradual compression) in high-risk cases.

SUGGESTED READINGS

Furfaro D, Stephens RS, Streiff MB, Brower R. Catheter-directed thrombolysis for intermediate-risk pulmonary embolism. *Ann Am Thorac Soc.* 2018;15(2):134–144.

Jaff MR, McMurtry MS, Archer SL, et al. Management of massive and submassive pulmonary embolism, iliofemoral deep vein thrombosis, and chronic thromboembolic pulmonary hypertension: a scientific statement from the American Heart Association. *Circulation.* 2011;123:1788–1830.

Abbreviations

CDT: Catheter-directed thrombolysis
CBC: Complete blood count
DVT: Deep vein thrombosis
IVC: Inferior vena cava
LV: Left ventricle
PE: Pulmonary embolism
RV: Right ventricle

Devices for Arrhythmia Detection, Management, and Prevention

• *Niel Shah, MD; Muhammad Saad, MD*

■ CASE PRESENTATION

A 75-year-old female patient with medical history of nonischemic heart failure with reduced ejection fraction (HFrEF) with left ventricular ejection fraction (LVEF) of 35%, hypertension, and diabetes mellitus presented with worsening shortness of breath on exertion and bilateral leg swelling. She had New York Heart Association (NYHA) functional class III symptoms. At home, she has been on optimal guideline-directed medical therapy (GDMT) consisting of valsartan-sacubitril, carvedilol, spironolactone, empagliflozin, and furosemide. She has been adherent with her all medications since the diagnosis of HFrEF was made 6 months ago.

On physical examination, blood pressure was 104/62 mmHg and pulse rate was 58 bpm. A grade 2/6 holosystolic murmur was heard at the apex, and a grade 1/6 crescendo-decrescendo systolic murmur was heard at the base. Bibasilar crackles, jugular venous distention, and significant bilateral lower extremity pitting edema were also present. Otherwise, the physical exam was unremarkable. Electrocardiogram showed sinus rhythm and left bundle branch block (LBBB) with QRS duration of 155 milliseconds. Laboratory studies were unremarkable except elevated B-type natriuretic peptide.

Echocardiogram showed an ejection fraction of 30%, elevated left ventricular filling pressures, mild to moderate mitral regurgitation, and mild aortic stenosis. The patient was started on intravenous furosemide to optimize her volume status. The heart failure team continued to follow her closely, and once euvolemia was achieved, she was planned for cardiac resynchronization therapy (CRT) implantation before the discharge since CRT is associated with improved LVEF, reduced symptoms, and improved survival rates in patients with LVEF less than 35%, NYHA functional class II to IV symptoms, and LBBB. The patient underwent CRT placement successfully before discharge, was followed up in the heart failure clinic after discharge, and reported improvement in her symptoms and exercise tolerance.

■ KEY POINTS

- Pacemakers provide appropriate heart rate response for cardiac functioning and hemodynamic effects.
- Implantable cardioverter-defibrillator provides high-energy shock or antitachycardia therapy for termination of malignant arrhythmias.
- CRT improves cardiac dyssynchrony to help left ventricular function.

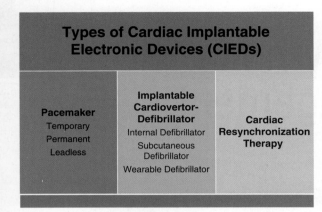

Types of Cardiac Implantable Electronic Devices (CIEDs)

Pacemaker
Temporary
Permanent
Leadless

Implantable Cardiovertor-Defibrillator
Internal Defibrillator
Subcutaneous Defibrillator
Wearable Defibrillator

Cardiac Resynchronization Therapy

FIGURE 8-1. Types of CIED.

■ INTRODUCTION

Cardiac implantable electronic devices (CIEDs) are specialized treatment for detection and treatment of tachy- or bradyarrhythmias. This chapter addresses the knowledge about use, indications, and complications associated with CIEDs.

■ CARDIAC PACEMAKERS

Cardiac pacemakers are effective treatments for a variety of bradyarrhythmias by providing appropriate heart rate response to reestablish effective circulation. Pacemakers are mechanical devices that generate electrical impulses propagated via 1 or more pacing wires to promote the regular contraction of the atria and/or the ventricles. They can be temporary or permanent.

Mechanism of Action

The pacemaker senses electrical signals from cardiac chambers and responds by inhibiting or triggering pacing. Various programming algorithms allow further control of pacing mode and rate. Most modern pacemakers capture and store a breadth of information, such as event counts, heart rate histograms, and electrograms of atrial and ventricular arrhythmia episodes that can further guide management, follow-up, and troubleshooting. Different types/modes of pacemakers, such as single-chamber pacemakers, dual-chamber pacemakers, rate-adaptive pacemakers, cardiac resynchronization therapy pacemaker (CRTp)/cardiac resynchronization therapy defibrillator (CRTd), and leadless pacemakers, are used depending on the underlying conduction abnormalities and needs of the patients. Leadless pacemakers are discussed briefly in a separate section.

Indications and Contraindications for Pacing

Generally, pacing is indicated when symptomatic bradycardias ensue. Cardiac electrical signaling can be disrupted by diseases of the sinus node, atrioventricular (AV) node, or His-Purkinje system due to aging, fibrosis, inflammation, infarction, or other conditions. It is preferred to consider temporary pacing when bradyarrhythmia is reversible. The type of pacemaker (atrial, ventricular, dual-chamber, or biventricular) is usually determined by the nature of the conduction system defect (sinus node, AV node, or intraventricular conduction delay). The indications for temporary and permanent pacing are as follows:

1. Temporary pacing
   - Temporary pacemaker implantation after ST-segment elevation myocardial infarction is recommended if symptomatic bradyarrhythmia is unresponsive to medical treatment (American College of Cardiology Foundation [ACCF]/American Heart Association [AHA]/Heart Rhythm Society [HRS] class I, level C) or as a prophylactic therapy in patients with high-grade AV block and/or new bundle branch or bifascicular block in patients with anterior/lateral myocardial infarction.
   - Temporary pacing after cardiac surgery may be required in patients with symptomatic bradyarrhythmias that occur after cardiac surgery.

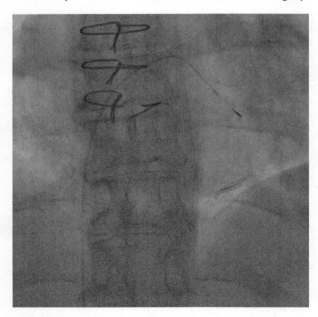

FIGURE 8-2. Temporary pacemaker used in ST-segment elevation myocardial infarction.

If symptomatic complete AV block or severe sick sinus syndrome lasts more than 5 to 7 days after cardiac surgery, then permanent pacemaker is usually implanted.

- Temporary pacing for AV block associated with Lyme disease (Lyme carditis) may be required for patients with advanced AV block (Infectious Diseases Society of America grade B-III).

2. Permanent pacing
   - ACCF/AHA/HRS recommendations for permanent pacing in patients with sick sinus syndrome are outlined in Table 8-1.

■ **TABLE 8-1. Recommendations for Permanent Pacing in Sinus Node Dysfunction (SND) (Level of Evidence: C)**

Class I: Permanent pacemaker implantation is indicated for
1. SND with documented symptomatic bradycardia, including frequent sinus pauses that produce symptoms. (Level of Evidence: C)
2. Symptomatic chronotropic incompetence. (Level of Evidence: C)
3. Symptomatic sinus bradycardia that results from required drug therapy for medical conditions. (Level of Evidence: C)

Class IIa: Permanent pacemaker implantation is reasonable for
1. Syncope of unexplained origin when clinically significant abnormalities of sinus node function are discovered or provoked in electrophysiological studies. (Level of Evidence: C)
2. SND with heart rate <40 bpm when a clear association between significant symptoms consistent with bradycardia and the actual presence of bradycardia has not been documented. (Level of Evidence: C)

Class IIb: Permanent pacemaker implantation may be considered in
1. Minimally symptomatic patients with chronic heart rate <40 bpm while awake. (Level of Evidence: C)

Class III: Permanent pacemaker implantation is not indicated in
1. SND in asymptomatic patients. (Level of Evidence: C)
2. SND in patients for whom the symptoms suggestive of bradycardia have been clearly documented to occur in the absence of bradycardia. (Level of Evidence: C)
3. SND with symptomatic bradycardia due to nonessential drug therapy. (Level of Evidence: C)

- ACCF/AHA/HRS recommendations for permanent pacing in patients with AV node dysfunction are outlined in Table 8-2.
- ACCF/AHA/HRS recommendations for permanent pacing in chronic bifascicular block are outlined in Table 8-3.
- ACCF/AHA/HRS recommendations for permanent pacing after the acute phase of myocardial infarction are outlined in Table 8-4.
- ACCF/AHA/HRS recommendations for permanent pacing in hypersensitive carotid sinus syndrome and neurocardiogenic syncope are outlined in Table 8-5.
- ACCF/AHA/HRS recommendations for pacing after cardiac transplantation are outlined in Table 8-6.
- ACCF/AHA/HRS recommendations for permanent pacemakers that automatically detect and pace to terminate tachycardias are outlined in Table 8-7.
- ACCF/AHA/HRS recommendations for pacing to prevent tachycardia are outlined in Table 8-8.
- ACCF/AHA/HRS recommendation for pacing to prevent atrial fibrillation are outlined in Table 8-9.
- ACCF/AHA/HRS recommendations for pacing in patients with hypertrophic cardiomyopathy are outlined in Table 8-10.
- ACCF/AHA/HRS recommendations for permanent pacing in children, adolescents, and patients with congenital heart disease are outlined in Table 8-11.

Equipment

Permanent pacemaker consists of:

- Implantable pulse generator: Source of energy with battery
- Leads: Generally, 2 leads that conduct electric current to the myocardium

Procedure

- The generator is usually implanted in left or right pectoral region, and the leads are introduced to pacing chamber via subclavian or axillary veins via standard puncture (Seldinger technique) or cephalic vein or subclavian vein via cut down.
- A pocket is formed in subcutaneous tissue at the infraclavicular level by using a scalpel, and the generator can be positioned.

■ TABLE 8-2. Recommendations for Pacing in Acquired AV Conduction Abnormalities

Class I: Permanent pacemaker implantation is indicated for
1. Third-degree and advanced second-degree AV block at any anatomic level associated with bradycardia with symptoms (including heart failure) or ventricular arrhythmias presumed to be due to AV block. (Level of Evidence: C)
2. Third-degree and advanced second-degree AV block at any anatomic level associated with arrhythmias and other medical conditions that require drug therapy that results in symptomatic bradycardia. (Level of Evidence: C)
3. Third-degree and advanced second-degree AV block at any anatomic level in awake, symptom-free patients in sinus rhythm, with documented periods of asystole ≥3.0 seconds or any escape rate <40 bpm, or with an escape rhythm that is below the AV node. (Level of Evidence: C)
4. Third-degree and advanced second-degree AV block at any anatomic level in awake, symptom-free patients with AF and bradycardia with 1 or more pauses of at least 5 seconds or longer. (Level of Evidence: C)
5. Third-degree and advanced second-degree AV block at any anatomic level after catheter ablation of the AV junction. (Level of Evidence: C)
6. Third-degree and advanced second-degree AV block at any anatomic level associated with postoperative AV block that is not expected to resolve after cardiac surgery. (Level of Evidence: C)
7. Third-degree and advanced second-degree AV block at any anatomic level associated with neuromuscular diseases with AV block, such as myotonic muscular dystrophy, Kearns-Sayre syndrome, Erb dystrophy (limb-girdle muscular dystrophy), and peroneal muscular atrophy, with or without symptoms. (Level of Evidence: B)
8. Second-degree AV block with associated symptomatic bradycardia regardless of type or site of block. (Level of Evidence: B)
9. Asymptomatic persistent third-degree AV block at any anatomic site with average awake ventricular rates of 40 bpm or faster if cardiomegaly or LV dysfunction is present or if the site of block is below the AV node. (Level of Evidence: B)
10. Second- or third-degree AV block during exercise in the absence of myocardial ischemia. (Level of Evidence: C)

Class IIa: Permanent pacemaker implantation is reasonable for
1. Persistent third-degree AV block with an escape rate >40 bpm in asymptomatic adult patients without cardiomegaly. (Level of Evidence: C)
2. Asymptomatic second-degree AV block at intra- or infra-His levels found at electrophysiologic study. (Level of Evidence: B)
3. First- or second-degree AV block with symptoms similar to those of pacemaker syndrome or hemodynamic compromise. (Level of Evidence: B)
4. Asymptomatic type II second-degree AV block with a narrow QRS. When type II second-degree AV block occurs with a wide QRS, including isolated right bundle branch block, pacing becomes a Class I recommendation. (Level of Evidence: B)

Class IIb: Permanent pacemaker implantation may be considered for
1. Neuromuscular diseases such as myotonic muscular dystrophy, Erb dystrophy (limb-girdle muscular dystrophy), and peroneal muscular atrophy with any degree of AV block (including first-degree AV block), with or without symptoms, because there may be unpredictable progression of AV conduction disease. (Level of Evidence: B)
2. AV block in the setting of drug use and/or drug toxicity when the block is expected to recur even after the drug is withdrawn. (Level of Evidence: B)

Class III: Permanent pacemaker implantation is not indicated in
1. Asymptomatic first-degree AV block. (Level of Evidence: B)
2. Asymptomatic type I second-degree AV block at the supra-His (AV node) level or that which is not known to be intra- or infra-Hisian. (Level of Evidence: C)
3. AV block that is expected to resolve and is unlikely to recur (e.g., drug toxicity, Lyme disease, or transient increases in vagal tone or during hypoxia in sleep apnea syndrome in the absence of symptoms). (Level of Evidence: B)

■ **TABLE 8-3. Recommendations for Permanent Pacing in Chronic Bifascicular Block**

Class I: Permanent pacemaker implantation is indicated for
1. Advanced second-degree AV block or intermittent third-degree AV block. (Level of Evidence: B)
2. Type II second-degree AV block. (Level of Evidence: B)
3. Alternating bundle branch block. (Level of Evidence: C)

Class IIa: Permanent pacemaker implantation is reasonable for
1. Syncope not demonstrated to be due to AV block when other likely causes have been excluded, specifically ventricular tachycardia (VT). (Level of Evidence: B)
2. An incidental finding at electrophysiologic study of a markedly prolonged His ventricular (HV) interval (≥100 milliseconds) in asymptomatic patients.
3. An incidental finding at electrophysiologic study of pacing-induced infra-His block that is not physiologic. (Level of Evidence: B)

Class IIb: Permanent pacemaker implantation may be considered in the setting of
1. Neuromuscular diseases such as myotonic muscular dystrophy, Erb dystrophy (limb-girdle muscular dystrophy), and peroneal muscular atrophy with bifascicular block or any fascicular block, with or without symptoms. (Level of Evidence: C)

Class III: Permanent pacemaker implantation is not indicated for
1. Fascicular block without AV block or symptoms. (Level of Evidence: B)
2. Fascicular block with first-degree AV block without symptoms. (Level of Evidence: B)

■ **TABLE 8-4. Recommendations for Permanent Pacing After the Acute Phase of Myocardial Infarction**

Class I: Permanent ventricular pacing is indicated for
1. Persistent second-degree AV block in the His-Purkinje system with alternating bundle branch block or third-degree AV block within or below the His-Purkinje system after ST-segment elevation myocardial infarction. (Level of Evidence: B)
2. Transient advanced second- or third-degree infranodal AV block and associated bundle branch block. If the site of block is uncertain, an electrophysiologic study may be necessary. (Level of Evidence: B)
3. Persistent and symptomatic second- or third-degree AV block. (Level of Evidence: C)

Class IIb: Permanent ventricular pacing may be considered for
1. Persistent second- or third-degree AV block at the AV node level, even in the absence of symptoms. (Level of Evidence: B)

Class III: Permanent ventricular pacing is not indicated for
1. Transient AV block in the absence of intraventricular conduction defects. (Level of Evidence: B)
2. Transient AV block in the presence of isolated left anterior fascicular block. (Level of Evidence: B)
3. New bundle branch block or fascicular block in the absence of AV block. (Level of Evidence: B)
4. Persistent asymptomatic first-degree AV block in the presence of bundle branch or fascicular block. (Level of Evidence: B)

- Over the guidewire, leads are delivered using a peelable sheath.
- The leads are fixed in the myocardium after parameter check.
- Final testing can be done after generator positioning in the pocket before closing with sutures.

Leadless Pacemakers

The Micra transcatheter pacing system leadless pacemaker is US Food and Drug Administration approved for use in patients with atrial fibrillation or other arrhythmias including bradycardia-tachycardia syndrome (Figure 8-4). It is 90% smaller than a transvenous pacemaker. The efficacy is based on a clinical trial in 719 patients that showed adequate pacing capture threshold in 98% of patients 6 months after implantation. The device is implanted via a femoral vein transcatheter approach. The primary advantage of a leadless pacemaker is the elimination of several complications associated with transvenous pacemakers and leads such as pocket infections, hematoma, lead dislodgment, and lead fracture. The leadless pacemaker also has cosmetic appeal because there is no chest incision or visible pacemaker pocket. However, leadless pacemakers provide only single-chamber ventricular pacing (right ventricle) and lack defibrillation capacity. Battery life is approximately 5 to 15 years, which is comparable to that of a transvenous pacemaker. Complications may occur related to femoral vein access or need for device repositioning, and there is a moderate risk of cardiac perforation with subsequent pericardial effusion.

■ **TABLE 8-5. Recommendations for Permanent Pacing in Hypersensitive Carotid Sinus Syndrome and Neurocardiogenic Syncope**

Class I: Permanent pacing is indicated for
1. Recurrent syncope caused by spontaneously occurring carotid sinus stimulation and carotid sinus pressure that induces ventricular asystole of >3 seconds. (Level of Evidence: C)

Class IIa: Permanent pacing is reasonable for
1. Syncope without clear, provocative events and with a hypersensitive cardioinhibitory response of 3 seconds or longer. (Level of Evidence: C)

Class IIb: Permanent pacing may be considered for
1. Significantly symptomatic neurocardiogenic syncope associated with bradycardia documented spontaneously or at the time of tilt-table testing. (Level of Evidence: B)

Class III: Permanent pacing is not indicated for
1. A hypersensitive cardioinhibitory response to carotid sinus stimulation without symptoms or with vague symptoms. (Level of Evidence: C)
2. Situational vasovagal syncope in which avoidance behavior is effective and preferred. (Level of Evidence: C)

■ **TABLE 8-6. Recommendations for Pacing After Cardiac Transplantation**

Class I: Permanent pacing is indicated for
1. Persistent inappropriate or symptomatic bradycardia not expected to resolve and for other Class I indications for permanent pacing. (Level of Evidence: C)

Class IIb: Permanent pacing may be considered
1. When relative bradycardia is prolonged or recurrent, which limits rehabilitation or discharge after postoperative recovery from cardiac transplantation. (Level of Evidence: C)
2. For syncope after cardiac transplantation even when bradyarrhythmia has not been documented. (Level of Evidence: C)

■ **TABLE 8-7. Recommendations for Permanent Pacemakers That Automatically Detect and Pace to Terminate Tachycardias**

Class IIa: Permanent pacing is reasonable for
1. Symptomatic recurrent SVT that is reproducibly terminated by pacing when catheter ablation and/or drugs fail to control the arrhythmia or produce intolerable side effects. (Level of Evidence: C)

Class III: Permanent pacing is not indicated
1. In the presence of an accessory pathway that has the capacity for rapid anterograde conduction. (Level of Evidence: C)

■ **TABLE 8-8. Recommendations for Pacing to Prevent Tachycardia**

Class I: Permanent pacing is indicated for
1. Sustained pause-dependent VT, with or without QT prolongation. (Level of Evidence: C)

Class IIa: Permanent pacing is reasonable for
1. High-risk patients with congenital long-QT syndrome. (Level of Evidence: C)

Class IIb: Permanent pacing may be considered for
1. Prevention of symptomatic, drug-refractory, recurrent atrial fibrillation in patients with coexisting sinus node dysfunction. (Level of Evidence: B)

Class III: Permanent pacing is not indicated for
1. Frequent or complex ventricular ectopic activity without sustained VT in the absence of the long-QT syndrome. (Level of Evidence: C)
2. Torsade de pointes VT due to reversible causes. (Level of Evidence: A)

■ **TABLE 8-9. Recommendation for Pacing to Prevent Atrial Fibrillation**

Class III: Permanent pacing is not indicated for the prevention of atrial fibrillation in patients without any other indication for pacemaker implantation. (Level of Evidence: B)

■ **TABLE 8-10.** Recommendations for Pacing in Patients With Hypertrophic Cardiomyopathy

Class I: Permanent pacing is indicated for
1. Sinus node dysfunction or AV block in patients with hypertrophic cardiomyopathy (HCM) (Level of Evidence: C)

Class IIa: Permanent pacing may be considered
1. In medically refractory symptomatic patients with HCM and significant resting or provoked LV outflow tract obstruction. (Level of Evidence: A)

Class III: Permanent pacemaker implantation is not indicated for
1. Patients who are asymptomatic or whose symptoms are medically controlled. (Level of Evidence: C)
2. Symptomatic patients without evidence of LV outflow tract obstruction. (Level of Evidence: C)

■ **TABLE 8-11.** Recommendations for Permanent Pacing in Children, Adolescents, and Patients With Congenital Heart Disease

Class I: Permanent pacemaker implantation is indicated for
1. Advanced second- or third-degree AV block associated with symptomatic bradycardia, ventricular dysfunction, or low cardiac output. (Level of Evidence: C)
2. Sinus node dysfunction (SND) with correlation of symptoms during age-inappropriate bradycardia. The definition of bradycardia varies with the patient's age and expected heart rate. (Level of Evidence: B)
3. Postoperative advanced second- or third-degree AV block that is not expected to resolve or that persists at least 7 days after cardiac surgery. (Level of Evidence: B)
4. Congenital third-degree AV block with a wide QRS escape rhythm, complex ventricular ectopy, or ventricular dysfunction. (Level of Evidence: B)
5. Congenital third-degree AV block in the infant with a ventricular rate <55 bpm or with congenital heart disease and a ventricular rate <70 bpm. (Level of Evidence: C)

Class IIa: Permanent pacemaker implantation is reasonable for
1. Patients with congenital heart disease and sinus bradycardia for the prevention of recurrent episodes of intra-atrial reentrant tachycardia; SND may be intrinsic or secondary to antiarrhythmic treatment. (Level of Evidence: C)
2. Congenital third-degree AV block beyond the first year of life with an average heart rate <50 bpm, abrupt pauses in ventricular rate that are 2 or 3 times the basic cycle length, or associated with symptoms due to chronotropic incompetence. (Level of Evidence: B)
3. Sinus bradycardia with complex congenital heart disease with a resting heart rate <40 bpm or pauses in ventricular rate >3 seconds. (Level of Evidence: C)
4. Patients with congenital heart disease and impaired hemodynamics due to sinus bradycardia or loss of AV synchrony. (Level of Evidence: C)
5. Unexplained syncope in the patient with prior congenital heart surgery complicated by transient complete heart block with residual fascicular block after a careful evaluation to exclude other causes of syncope. (Level of Evidence: B)

CLASS IIb: Permanent pacemaker implantation may be considered for
1. Transient postoperative third-degree AV block that reverts to sinus rhythm with residual bifascicular block. (Level of Evidence: C)
2. Congenital third-degree AV block in asymptomatic children or adolescents with an acceptable rate, a narrow QRS complex, and normal ventricular function. (Level of Evidence: B)
3. Asymptomatic sinus bradycardia after biventricular repair of congenital heart disease with a resting heart rate <40 bpm or pauses in ventricular rate >3 seconds. (Level of Evidence: C)

Class III: Permanent pacemaker implantation is not indicated for
1. Transient postoperative AV block with return of normal AV conduction in the otherwise asymptomatic patient. (Level of Evidence: B)
2. Asymptomatic bifascicular block with or without first-degree AV block after surgery for congenital heart disease in the absence of prior transient complete AV block. (Level of Evidence: C)
3. Asymptomatic type I second-degree AV block. (Level of Evidence: C)
4. Asymptomatic sinus bradycardia with the longest relative risk interval <3 seconds and a minimum heart rate >40 bpm. (Level of Evidence: C)

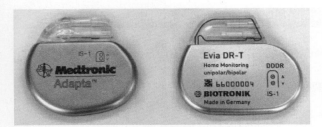

FIGURE 8-3. Cardiac pacemaker pulse generators.

■ IMPLANTABLE CARDIOVERTER-DEFIBRILLATOR

An implantable cardioverter-defibrillator (ICD) is a battery-powered device that can detect malignant arrhythmias and is capable of aborting them by providing energy. It was first successfully placed in 1980 and since then has revolutionized the world of cardiology.

Mechanism of Action

The ICD system consists of a pulse generator, pacing/sensing electrodes, and defibrillation electrodes. The pulse generator (Figure 8-5) contains the sensing circuitry, the high-voltage capacitors, and the battery. The pulse generator is usually placed in the infraclavicular region of the anterior chest (prepectoral or subpectoral). The impulses generated are transmitted to the myocardium via transvenous leads. The contemporary epicardial systems are still available and may be necessary as a result of anatomic limitations to placing a transvenous lead(s). In addition, a subcutaneous ICD system is available in which the pulse generator is placed overlying the left lower lateral ribs (Figure 8-5). A pulse generator will last for 5 or more years in most patients.

Pacing and sensing functions require a pair of electrodes. Contemporary pacemakers and defibrillators usually use bipolar ventricular leads, which provide accurate sensing, with high amplitude and narrow electrograms. Additionally, bipolar leads reduce the risk of extraneous interference, which could lead to inappropriate device function (inappropriate shocks). The defibrillation function of the electrodes requires a relatively large surface area and positioning of the lead to maximize the density of current flow through the ventricular myocardium. Contemporary ICD systems use a coil of wire that extends along the ventricular lead as the primary defibrillation electrode. Thus, a single transvenous lead can accomplish

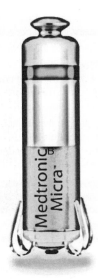

A

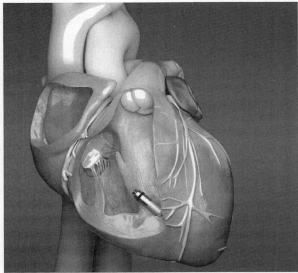

B

FIGURE 8-4. A, B. Leadless pacemaker. The blue arrow shows the implanted leadless pacemaker. (See color insert.)

all pacing, sensing, and defibrillation functions. Additional defibrillation electrodes improve defibrillation efficacy and reduce the defibrillation threshold. Most contemporary ICD systems have 2 or 3 defibrillation electrodes. There are 3 types of pacing offered by current transvenous systems. Single-chamber systems have only a

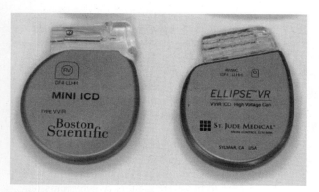

FIGURE 8-5. ICD pulse generators.

right ventricular (RV) lead. Dual-chamber systems have right atrial (RA) and RV leads. Cardiac resynchronization therapy (CRT; also called biventricular) systems have RA, RV, and left ventricular (LV) leads or, in some patients with permanent atrial fibrillation, RV and LV leads.

Indications

Main indications for ICD use include primary and secondary prevention of sudden cardiac death (SCD). It is indicated for **primary prevention of SCD** in patients who remain high risk for ventricular tachycardia (VT)/ventricular fibrillation (VF) after the use of optimal medical management, such as:

- Patients with heart failure with reduced ejection fraction (HFrEF) with LV ejection fraction (LVEF) of 35% or lower and with New York Heart Association (NYHA) functional class II to III after 3 months of guideline-directed medical therapy (GDMT)

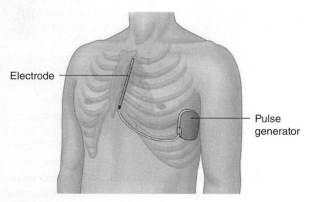

FIGURE 8-6. Subcutaneous ICD.

- Patients with a prior myocardial infarction (at least 40 days ago) and LVEF of 30% or lower
- Patients with congenital long QT syndrome who have recurrent symptoms and/or torsades de pointes despite medical therapy
- High-risk patients with Brugada syndrome, catecholaminergic polymorphic VT, and other channelopathies
- High-risk patients with hypertrophic cardiomyopathy

An ICD implantation is recommended for the **secondary prevention of SCD** in patients with prior sustained VT or VF or resuscitated SCD thought to be due to VT/VF.

Contraindications

ICD implantation is not recommended in the following patients:

- Patients with ventricular tachyarrhythmias due to a transient or completely reversible disorder in the absence of structural heart disease (eg, electrolyte imbalance, drugs, hypoxia, acute myocardial infarction, sepsis, drowning, electric shock, or trauma)
- Patients with incessant VT or VF in whom other therapies (eg, catheter ablation) should be considered first
- Patients with end-stage heart failure refractory to optimal medical treatment and not candidates for heart transplantation
- Patients with VT or VF in whom risk of SCD normalized after successful ablation

Equipment and Procedure

Equipment consists of the following:

- Generator: Contains battery
- Header and can: Titanium structure for electrical circuitry
- Leads: Has coil at the distal tip for energy transmission

■ CARDIAC RESYNCHRONIZATION THERAPY

Many patients with LV dysfunction have additional interventricular or intraventricular dyssynchrony, which can further impair cardiac output. CRT targets and treats ventricular dyssynchrony and has been associated with reduced heart failure hospitalization, improved functional status, better quality of life, and decreased mortality in multiple randomized controlled trials.

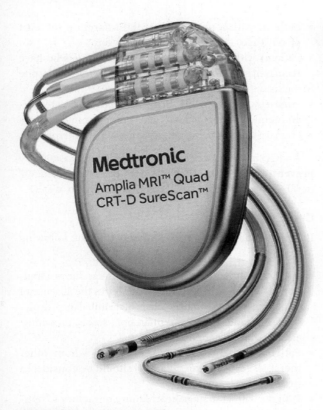

FIGURE 8-7. Example of CRT.

Mechanism of Action

The predominant mechanism of action of CRT is ventricular resynchronization in addition to its ability to function as ICD. CRT also improves LV filling (preload) by shortening effective AV delay to a more optimal value. CRT usually consists of 3 leads: RA lead, RV lead, and LV lead. The routine delivery of CRT is via the coronary sinus in conjunction with endocardial RV and RA leads (Figure 8-7).

Indications and Contraindications

ACCF/AHA/HRS recommendations for CRT are outlined in Table 8-12.

■ WEARABLE CARDIOVERTER-DEFIBRILLATOR

There are some situations when ICD implantation is not immediately feasible, may be of uncertain benefit, or may not be covered by third-party payers or when an ICD

■ **TABLE 8-12. Recommendations for Cardiac Resynchronization Therapy**

Class I: CRT is indicated for
1. Patients who have LVEF ≤35%, sinus rhythm, LBBB with a QRS duration ≥150 ms, and NYHA class II, III, or ambulatory IV symptoms on GDMT. (Level of Evidence: A for NYHA class III/IV; Level of Evidence: B for NYHA class II)

Class IIa: CRT can be useful for
1. Patients who have LVEF ≤35%, sinus rhythm, LBBB with a QRS duration 120-149 ms, and NYHA class II, III, or ambulatory IV symptoms on GDMT. (Level of Evidence: B)
2. Patients who have LVEF ≤35%, sinus rhythm, a non-LBBB pattern with a QRS duration ≥150 ms, and NYHA class III/ambulatory class IV symptoms on GDMT. (Level of Evidence: A)
3. Patients with atrial fibrillation and LVEF ≤35% on GDMT if (a) the patient requires ventricular pacing or otherwise meets CRT criteria and (b) AV nodal ablation or pharmacologic rate control will allow near 100% ventricular pacing with CRT. (Level of Evidence: B)
4. Patients on GDMT who have LVEF ≤35% and are undergoing new or replacement device placement with anticipated requirement for significant (>40%) ventricular pacing. (Level of Evidence: C)

Class IIb: CRT may be considered for
1. Patients who have LVEF ≤30%, ischemic etiology of heart failure, sinus rhythm, LBBB with a QRS duration of ≥150 ms, and NYHA class I symptoms on GDMT. (Level of Evidence: C)
2. Patients who have LVEF ≤35%, sinus rhythm, a non-LBBB pattern with QRS duration 120-149 ms, and NYHA class III/ambulatory class IV on GDMT. (Level of Evidence: B)
3. Patients who have LVEF ≤35%, sinus rhythm, a non-LBBB pattern with a QRS duration ≥150 ms, and NYHA class II symptoms on GDMT. (Level of Evidence: B)

Class III: CRT is not recommended for
1. Patients with NYHA class I or II symptoms and non-LBBB pattern with QRS duration <150 ms. (Level of Evidence: B)
2. Patients whose comorbidities and/or frailty limit survival with good functional capacity to <1 year. (Level of Evidence: C)

must be removed. In such cases, a wearable cardioverter-defibrillator (WCD; Life Vest) offers an alternative approach for the prevention of SCD (Figure 8-8). The WCD is an external device capable of automatic detection and defibrillation of VT and VF. The indications for considering WCD include the following:

- Patients with LVEF of 35% or lower who have had a myocardial infarction within the past 40 days
- Patients with LVEF of 35% or lower who have undergone coronary revascularization with coronary artery bypass graft surgery in the past 3 months
- Patients with newly diagnosed nonischemic cardiomyopathy with LVEF of 35% or lower that is potentially reversible
- Patients with a permanent ICD that must be explanted or those with a delay in implanting a newly indicated ICD (eg, due to systemic infection)
- Patients with severe heart failure who are awaiting heart transplantation

WCDs are very effective but also come with some limitations. The device will not be a good fit for some patients due to body habitus. Because it is an external device, it does not allow for pacemaker functionality. Also, patient interaction and compliance are very important for its functionality. There is also a risk of external noise leading to inappropriate shocks. Additionally, the device needs to be removed for bathing, and no protection is afforded while the device is off. Comfort may also be an issue for some patients due to the size and weight of the device.

■ IMPLANTABLE LOOP RECORDER

The implantable loop recorder (ILR) is a subcutaneous device used for diagnosing heart rhythm disorders. It is usually implanted under local anesthesia subcutaneously with a battery life of about 36 months (Figure 8-9). It stores retrospective electrocardiogram recordings when activated by patient, bystander, or automatically. Indications for an ILR include the following:

- Early phase of evaluation in patients with recurrent syncope of uncertain origin (in absence of high-risk criteria) if high likelihood of recurrent event during battery longevity (European Society of Cardiology [ESC] class I, level A)
- High-risk patients when thorough evaluation did not find cause of syncope or lead to a specific treatment and no conventional indications for ICD for primary prevention of SCD or pacemaker indication (ESC class I, level A)
- Should be considered in patients with suspected or certain reflex syncope presenting with frequent or severe syncopal episodes (ESC class IIa, level B)

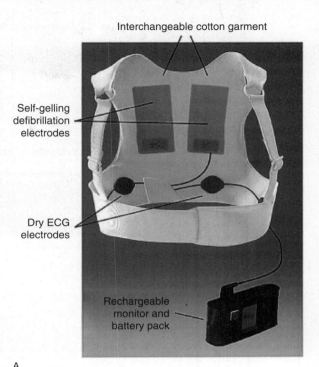

Interchangeable cotton garment

Self-gelling defibrillation electrodes

Dry ECG electrodes

Rechargeable monitor and battery pack

A

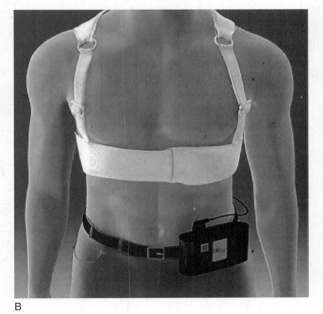

B

FIGURE 8-8. A, B. Wearable cardioverter defibrillator (Life Vest). (See color insert.)

Reveal LINQ (Medtronic, Minneapolis, USA)

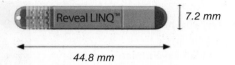

7.2 mm

44.8 mm

Reveal XT (Medtronic, Minneapolis, USA)

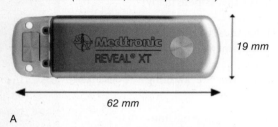

19 mm

62 mm

A

BioMonitor II (Biotronik SE & Co., Berlin, Germany)

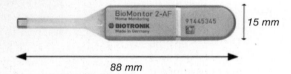

15 mm

88 mm

Confirm RX ICM (St. Jude Medical, Minnesota, USA)

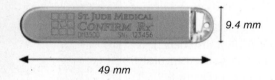

9.4 mm

49 mm

B

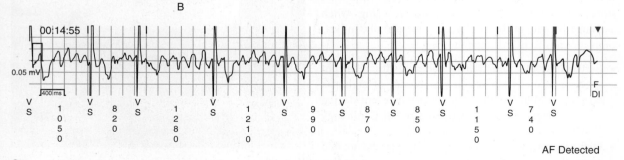

C

FIGURE 8-9. Examples of implantable loop recorder (**A, B**) and tracing (**C**) showing atrial fibrillation.

- May be considered in patients in whom epilepsy was previously suspected but treatment has proven ineffective (ESC class IIb, level B)
- May be considered in patients with unexplained falls (ESC class IIb, level B)

Despite potential clinical advantages and the recent technologic improvements in ILR, it is still underused in clinical practice. The ability to perform remote monitoring improves the diagnostic timing and the follow-up strategy for ILR patients with a potential reduction in healthcare costs. Additionally, the recent advent of injectable ILRs makes the procedure even easier.

■ COMPLICATIONS OF CIED IMPLANTATION (TABLE 8-13)

The complications related to any CIED placement are somewhat similar and include infection at the implantation site or endovascular leads, pocket hematoma, pneumothorax/hemothorax, lead displacement, cardiac tamponade, cardiac perforation (rare), tricuspid regurgitation, venous thrombosis and obstruction, generator failure, lead displacement, lead fracture, lead failure (undersensing or oversensing), and inappropriate shocks.

■ TROUBLESHOOTING

In patients with CIED, the HRS has recommended in-office evaluation 2 to 12 weeks after implantation, remote interrogation every 3 to 12 months, and in-person evaluation at least once every year.

Battery depletion: CIED malfunction may occur with battery depletion. Elective battery replacement indicator usually indicates that 90 days of reliable function are remaining, whereas end of life indicates a battery depleted to the point of unpredictable function.

Undersensing and oversensing: When the pacemaker fails to detect spontaneous myocardial depolarization and causes asynchronous pacing, this is known as undersensing. In such cases, atrial or ventricular pacing spikes arise regardless of P waves or QRS complex (Figure 8-10) and result in the appearance of too many pacing spikes on electrocardiogram. On the contrary, when the pacemaker senses electrical signals that it is not programmed to sense and results in inappropriate inhibition of the pacing stimulus, this is called oversensing (Figure 8-10). Usually in cases of undersensing or oversensing, lead sensitivity is adjusted to improve undersensing or oversensing. Some devices

■ TABLE 8-13. Summary of Complications of CIED Implantation	
Infection	Infection of the generator pocket or leads can occur at the time of CIED implantation or at any subsequent time. It can be life threatening, and complete removal of the CIED pulse generator and all leads with antibiotic therapy is strongly recommended for all patients. The use of an antibiotic-impregnated absorbable envelope at the time of CIED implantation has been shown to reduce major CIED infections in certain higher-risk populations.
Bleeding	Most patients undergoing transvenous CIED insertion have minimal blood loss or postoperative bleeding, but serious bleeding can sometimes occur. Patients who develop a significant pocket hematoma are at higher risk of developing device-related infection.
Cardiac perforation	Very rare complication but associated with significant morbidity and mortality.
Pneumothorax	Traditional subclavian access has a higher pneumothorax risk than the extrathoracic axillary vein micropuncture technique or cephalic vein access. The use of periprocedural venography to guide access can reduce the risk.
Lead malposition	Rare complication. If ventricular lead is placed into the atrial port and vice versa, then it can lead to pacemaker syndrome and LV systolic dysfunction. Inadvertent lead malposition in the left heart can be avoided intraoperatively by evaluating the paced QRS morphology in V1 or its equivalent, visualizing a guidewire going below the diaphragm and imaging in both the right and left anterior oblique projections.
Lead displacement and lead fracture	Usually, most lead dislodgements occur within first 3 months of implantation; in contrast, lead fractures can continue to occur during the follow-up period.

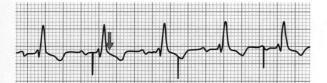

A. Showing undersensing after 3rd beat (blue arrow).

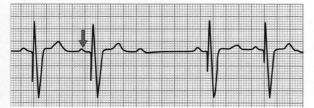

B. Showing oversensing. After the 3rd sinus P wave, pacing spike is absent (blue arrow).

FIGURE 8-10. A. Showing undersensing after third beat (blue arrow). **B.** Showing oversensing. After the third sinus P wave, pacing spike is absent (blue arrow).

can automatically adjust sensitivity based on the measured amplitude of sensed events.

Device-related arrhythmias: Two commonly encountered device-related arrhythmias due to pacemaker are pacemaker-mediated tachycardia (PMT) and upper rate behavior resulting in high or low ventricular rates. PMT is a sustained endless-loop tachycardia caused by the presence of the pacemaker. PMT is similar to a reentrant tachycardia, except that the pacemaker forms part of the reentrant circuit. The tachycardia could therefore be avoided by programming a sufficiently long postventricular atrial refractory period (PVARP). In addition, PMT can be terminated by magnet application, which changes the pacemaker mode to dual chamber. Upper-rate behavior is usually seen in dual-chambered pacemakers programmed to an atrial tracking mode as the atrial rate increases and approaches a certain upper threshold. Undesirable upper-rate

behavior is avoided by meticulous attention to intervals, by programming to allow a Wenckebach interval between the maximum tracking rate and the 2:1 block rate, and by allowing rate-adaptive shortening of the AV and PVARP intervals.

Inappropriate mode switches: Inappropriate mode switches can occasionally result in inappropriate detection and classification of events as atrial fibrillation. It is imperative to evaluate electrograms before therapeutic interventions for management of atrial arrhythmias.

Inappropriate shocks: Sometimes the ICD detects an unshockable rhythm such as atrial tachycardias and gives an inappropriate shock. Atrial fibrillation is the most common cause of inappropriate shock, followed by sinus tachycardia, atrial flutter, and atrial tachycardia. In patients who have received inappropriate ICD shocks for supraventricular tachycardia, device programming can be very helpful by turning supraventricular tachycardia discriminators on. In addition, optimizing ICDs to the individual patient's characteristics and adjusting therapy zones and detection intervals to more aggressive levels can significantly reduce the risk of recurrent shocks.

Failure to shock: The most common cause for failure to deliver shock is lead failure or programming the rate detection zone too high. In addition, lead malposition, dislodgement, fracture, or battery depletion should be considered as causes for failure to shock in the appropriate settings.

■ FUTURE DIRECTIONS

- Efforts have been ongoing to improve CIEDs to reduce risk of infection either by extracardiac implantation or improving the lead synthesis.
- Algorithms for improving sensing are being devised, especially in heart failure patients, to improve outcomes.

SUGGESTED READINGS

Epstein AE, DiMarco JP, Ellenbogen KA, et al; American College of Cardiology Foundation, American Heart Association Task Force on Practice Guidelines, Heart Rhythm Society. 2012 ACCF/AHA/HRS focused update incorporated into the ACCF/AHA/HRS 2008 guidelines for device-based therapy of cardiac rhythm abnormalities: a report of the American College of Cardiology Foundation/

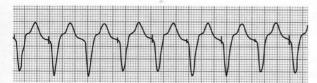

FIGURE 8-11. Example of pacemaker-mediated tachycardia (PMT).

American Heart Association Task Force on Practice Guidelines and the Heart Rhythm Society. *J Am Coll Cardiol.* 2013;61(3):e6-75.

Gillis AM, Russo AM, Ellenbogen KA, et al. Heart Rhythm Society, American College of Cardiology Foundation. HRS/ACCF expert consensus statement on pacemaker device and mode selection. Developed in partnership between the Heart Rhythm Society (HRS) and the American College of Cardiology Foundation (ACCF) and in collaboration with the Society of Thoracic Surgeons. *Heart Rhythm.* 2012;9(8):1344–1365.

Abbreviations

ACCF: American College of Cardiology Foundation
AHA: American Heart Association
AV: Atrioventricular
CRT: Cardiac resynchronization therapy
CIED: Cardiac implantable electronic device

ESC: European Society of Cardiology
GDMT: Guideline-directed medical therapy
HFrEF: Heart failure with reduced ejection fraction
HRS: Heart Rhythm Society
ICD: Implantable cardioverter-defibrillator
ILR: Implantable loop recorder
LBBB: Left bundle branch block
LV: Left ventricular
LVEF: Left ventricular ejection fraction
NYHA: New York Heart Association
PMT: Pacemaker-mediated tachycardia
PVARP: Postventricular atrial refractory period
RA: Right atrial
RV: Right ventricular
SCD: Sudden cardiac death
VT: Ventricular tachycardia
VF: Ventricular fibrillation
WCD: Wearable cardioverter-defibrillator

Respiratory Support Devices

• *Arundhati Dileep, MD*

■ CASE PRESENTATION

A 65-year-old woman with hypertension, diabetes mellitus, and asthma presented to the emergency department with the acute onset of shortness of breath. Over the prior 6 months, she has had 3 similar presentations. Each time, she has been admitted and treated with diuretics and bronchodilators, with improved symptoms. She follows up in clinic regularly.

On admission, her blood pressure is 156/88 mmHg and heart rate is 89 bpm. Her body mass index is 38 kg/m^2. She appears to be in respiratory distress. Her jugular venous pressure is not visible due to body habitus. She has diffuse crackles in the lungs with 2+ pitting edema.

Chest X-ray shows enlarged pulmonary arteries with bilateral infiltrates suggestive of pneumonia versus pulmonary edema. Echocardiography shows a small left ventricle with a sigmoid septum and an ejection fraction of 30%, borderline right ventricular dilatation, mild-moderate mitral regurgitation, and mild tricuspid regurgitation. Estimated right ventricular systolic pressure is 40 mmHg. She is started on intravenous furosemide and inhaled albuterol and ipratropium. Despite this treatment, she remains dyspneic, and subsequent laboratory studies reveal an increase in creatinine from 1.2 to 1.8 mg/dL. Her pro-B-type natriuretic peptide level was 1000 ng/dL. Blood gas showed pH of 7.10, PCO$_2$ of 70 mmHg, PaO$_2$ of 69 mmHg, and serum bicarbonate of 28 mmol/L. The patient was admitted to the coronary care unit for heart failure exacerbation and was initiated on bilevel positive airway pressure (BiPAP) for respiratory distress.

■ KEY POINTS

- In heart failure patients, BiPAP has been shown to improve symptom relief, intensive care unit and hospital length of stay, and ultimately quality of life.
- Coronary care unit physicians should familiarize themselves with respiratory devices used in day-to-day patient care.
- Mechanical ventilation has become sophisticated and is used to improve patient hemodynamics with less risk of lung injury.

■ TYPES OF RESPIRATORY SUPPORT DEVICES

In coronary care units, several devices are used for airway support and are considered vital components. They can be invasive or noninvasive depending on the clinical condition and patient's wishes.

Noninvasive Ventilation for Acute Respiratory Failure

Introduction

Noninvasive ventilation (NIV) avoids the use of endotracheal intubation and helps reduce the work of breathing

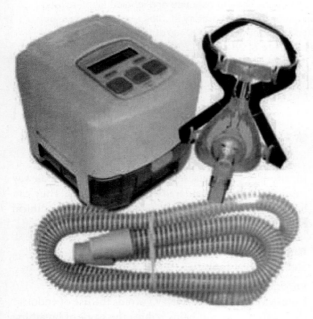

FIGURE 9-1. Types of respiratory devices.

Invasive devices
• Intubation and mechanical ventilation

Noninvasive devices
• CPAP/BiPAP
• High-flow nasal cannula

■ TABLE 9-1. Indications for BiPAP
Indications where NIV might be beneficial
Acute exacerbation of chronic obstructive pulmonary disease
Cardiogenic pulmonary edema
Postextubation respiratory failure
Postextubation in high-risk patients
Neuromuscular diseases
Acute asthma exacerbation
De novo respiratory failure
Immunocompromised adults
Obesity hypoventilation syndrome
Preoperative and postoperative cases
Scenarios where patients have a side status of do not resuscitate and do not intubate (palliative care)
Trauma
Pandemic viral illness

by offloading the respiratory muscles. It improves the alveolar gas exchange, improves the alveolar ventilation, and prevents the closure of the upper airway. It can be used via different interfaces, primarily face masks, oronasal face masks, or helmets.[1]

Literature Review

A Cochrane review included 14 randomized controlled trials comparing NIV plus usual care versus usual care alone. The use of NIV has shown a decreased need for intubation, with a relative risk (RR) of 0.41 (95% confidence interval [CI], 0.33-0.53). It has also been shown

to reduce mortality, with an RR of 0.52 (95% CI, 0.35-0.76), which results in a number needed to treat of 10 (95% CI, 7-20).[2,3]

Bilevel NIV (bilevel positive airway pressure [BiPAP]) has been shown to prevent intubation in patients with respiratory acidosis, as seen in our patient mentioned in the case. It has also been shown to reduce the rates of intubation, intensive care unit (ICU) and hospital length stay, and mortality.

Mechanism of Action

Bilevel NIV works as pressure-controlled ventilation leading to patent small airways moving pressurized air into the lungs. It works more during inspiration and reduces work in expiration to improve breathing discomfort. It can also be used as continuous pressure, called as continuous positive airway pressure (CPAP).

Equipment

BiPAP consists of a mask connected with tubing that is attached to a machine that blows air and has a console for parameter setup.

Indications and Contraindications

Major indications and contraindications of BiPAP use are listed in Tables 9-1 and 9-2.

Complications Associated With NIV

• Aspiration pneumonia
• Barotrauma
• Hemodynamic effects: hypotension and tachycardia

FIGURE 9-2. BiPAP machine.

■ TABLE 9-2. Contraindications of BiPAP	
Contraindications of NIV (Absolute)	**Contraindications of NIV (Relative)**
Cardiac or respiratory arrest	Uncooperative patient (agitation, confused)
Facial trauma	Inability to protect the airway
Facial burns	Excessive secretions
Upper airway obstruction	Impaired consciousness (GCS <8)
Multiorgan failure	Hemodynamic instability
Recent esophageal anastomosis	Acute pneumothorax
Coma	Vomiting
Arrhythmia with hemodynamic instability	

Abbreviation: GCS, Glasgow coma scale.

- Interface-related complications
- Facial skin lesions: erythema, pressure ulcers, and erythema
- Discomfort
- Claustrophobia
- Patient-ventilator dyssynchrony
- Rebreathing
- Air pressure– and flow-related complications
- Air leaks
- Nasal or oral dryness and nasal congestion
- Airway dryness
- Gastric insufflation

Monitoring and Troubleshooting

The patient must be closely monitored after being placed on NIV, and arterial blood gas sample must be obtained 30 minutes to 1 hour after the application of NIV to assess the effectiveness of the device in a particular clinical scenario.

Patients should be observed for altered sensorium, increasing respiratory distress, hemodynamic instability, copious secretions, vomiting, and refractory respiratory acidosis.

If any of these are observed, it is an indication of failure of NIV, and such a patient would require mechanical ventilation. If the patient is noted to have discomfort, air leak, dryness, or mucus plugging, then simple adjustments like mask size readjustments, decongestants, and humidification can be used to troubleshoot the problem.

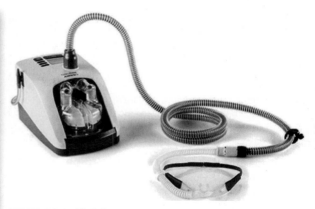

FIGURE 9-3. High-flow nasal cannula equipment.

High-Flow Nasal Cannula

Introduction

The first-line treatment for acute hypoxemic respiratory failure is supplemental oxygen. In the 2000s, high-flow nasal cannulas (HFNCs) gained attention as an alternative in such scenarios because it was less invasive compared to mechanical ventilation.

The differences between NIV and HFNC are the interfaces and the ability to provide consistent pressure versus different inspiratory and expiratory pressures. Whereas NIV interfaces add to the anatomic dead space, HFNC delivery decreases dead space. Because it is an open system, HFNC does not enhance the tidal volume like NIV.

Mechanism of Action

High flow rates lead to carbon dioxide washout, reduce the anatomic dead space, and reduce the work of breathing. The continuous high flow rates provide a degree of positive end-expiratory pressure (PEEP), which increases alveolar recruitment, reduces airflow resistance, and enhances oxygenation. The humidified gas reduces surface dehydration and improves secretion clearance, decreasing atelectasis.

Equipment

The HFNC system consists of a flow generator, active heated humidifier, single-limb heated circuit, and nasal cannula.

Through HFNC, flow rates as high as 60 L/min and higher oxygen concentrations (up to 100% FiO_2) can be provided to the patient. HFNC also provides a certain amount of PEEP.

Indications and Contraindications

The major indications and contraindications of HFNC use are listed in Tables 9-3 and 9-4.

■ TABLE 9-3. Indications for HFNC

Acute hypoxic respiratory failure
Postextubation respiratory failure
Postextubation in high-risk patients
Preintubation apneic oxygenation
Post–cardiac surgery respiratory failure
Scenarios where patients have a side status of do not resuscitate and do not intubate (palliative care)

Complications Associated With HFNC
Commonly, HFNC can be associated with local trauma, discomfort, epistaxis, abdominal distension, and barotrauma.

Monitoring and Troubleshooting

- Patients placed on HFNC must be closely monitored after 1 hour of application of the HFNC.
- It is essential to assess the respiratory rate oxygenation (ROX) index because this index helps assess the success of HFNC at 12 hours from ICU admission.
- ROX index = (SpO_2/FiO_2)/respiratory rate.
- An ROX index greater than or equal to 4.88 at 12 hours from the time of ICU admission was associated with a lower risk for mechanical ventilation even after adjusting for the other confounding variables. It has a positive predictive value of 89.4%.
- If there is a failure of HFNC, then patients might need intubation and mechanical ventilation.
- HFNC can be weaned once clinical status improves and oxygen saturation is maintained above 92%.
- For weaning purposes, FiO_2 can be reduced to a target of 40%, after which flow can be reduced to 30 L/min. Once the target is achieved, the patient can be transitioned to nasal cannula.

Mechanical Ventilation Through Endotracheal Intubation

Introduction
Mechanical ventilation (MV) is an invasive modality of positive-pressure ventilation that helps ventilate or oxygenate patients who cannot sustain the necessary level of ventilation to maintain adequate gas exchange.

Mechanism of Action
During a normal respiratory cycle of inspiration, the primary ventilatory muscles increase the size of the thoracic cavity, overcoming the elastic forces of the lungs and thorax and the resistance of the airways. As the volume increases, there is generation of negative intrathoracic pressure, which in turn leads to lung expansion. Gas flows from the atmosphere into the lungs due to the transpulmonary pressure gradient. During expiration, the inspiratory muscles relax. The elastic forces of the lung and thorax cause a decrease in volume, and as a result, exhalation occurs.

During ventilatory failure, the patient is unable to perform this task effectively. An invasive mechanical ventilator is a device that can fully or partially substitute for the ventilatory work performed by the patient's muscles.

The goals of MV include increasing lung volume by preventing atelectasis, improving gas exchange by maintaining ventilation and oxygenation, and reducing the work of breathing.

Equipment
Ventilator technology has evolved since the introduction of the Engstrom 100, the first volume-controlled mechanical ventilator in 1951. The current technology

■ TABLE 9-4. Contraindications of HFNC

Cardiac or respiratory arrest
Facial trauma
Facial burns
Upper airway obstruction
Uncooperative patients, reduced levels of consciousness
Hemodynamic instability

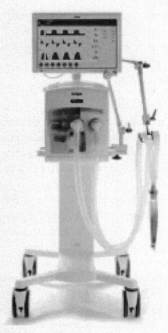

FIGURE 9-4. Mechanical ventilator equipment.

is controlled by a microprocessor-controlled pneumatic drive mechanism.

MV can be of primarily 2 types: an open-loop control circuit where the desired output is selected and the ventilator achieves the desired output without any further input from the clinician or the ventilator itself, or a closed-loop control circuit where the desired output is selected, the ventilator measures a specific parameter or variable (pressure, flow, or volume) continuously, and the input is constantly adjusted to match the desired output. This closed-loop system is also known as a servo-controlled system.

Indications
Indications for MV are listed in Table 9-5.

Contraindications
There are no major contraindications except pneumothorax and patient refusal.

Modes of MV
Different modes of MV work in different phases of the respiratory cycle. The trigger phase initiates a breath. When the ventilation is fully controlled, the trigger variable is time; thus, the breath is initiated at fixed intervals.

When the ventilator synchronizes the breath delivery with a signal related to the patient's effort, inspiration is initiated when a given flow or pressure decrease is noted by the ventilator. The target (or controlled) phase is the pressure or flow maintained until the inspiration ends.

The cycling phase determines the end of the inspiratory phase. A pressure, flow, or preset time can cycle the breath. When the variable reaches the preset value, the passive expiratory phase starts.

Breaths can therefore be fully controlled, trigger and cycling are time controlled, the target variable is reached passively, and the patient does not actively contribute to

■ TABLE 9-5. Indications for Invasive Mechanical Ventilation

Acute ventilatory failure: apnea, acute respiratory distress, metabolic acidosis, or refractory respiratory acidosis
Impending ventilatory failure: failure of NIV or HFNC
Acute hypoxemia respiratory failure
Neuromuscular diseases
Airway protection in postoperative patients
Smoke inhalation injury
Trauma
Refractory shock

the breath. A partially supported or assisted combination of ventilator assistance and patient effort occurs in the same cycle, and breathing is unassisted when the inspiratory flow is generated entirely by the patient's respiratory muscles.

Complications With Invasive MV
MV is a life-saving modality but is associated with some serious complications related to the cardiopulmonary system. Positive-pressure ventilation has hemodynamic effects through various heart-lung interactions. The high intrathoracic pressure can negatively impact the right ventricular afterload and function. Echocardiographic studies in patients with acute respiratory distress syndrome have reported a prevalence of acute cor pulmonale of about 22%.

Prolonged delirium is a complication associated with sedatives and neuromuscular blockade, which are used in patients on MV. Therefore, use of a sedation protocol and daily sedation interruption are important.

Oxygen toxicity is also a concern in the early days of MV. It is associated with increased vascular resistance; it can decrease the parasympathetic drive and hence decrease cardiac output. It is also associated with vasoconstrictive effects on cerebral and coronary perfusion.

MV can be associated with respiratory muscle dysfunction and weaning difficulties. There is increased risk of critical illness myopathy or polyneuropathy associated with prolonged MV. MV is also associated with an increased risk of ventilator-acquired pneumonia due to increased micro-aspiration from the oropharyngeal cavity and impaired mucociliary clearance. This can be mitigated by limiting the sedation and shortening the duration of MV.

MV can also cause ventilator-induced lung injury, including volutrauma, barotrauma, and atelectotrauma.

Finally, MV is associated with some long-term sequelae, including postintensive syndrome, which could include functional disabilities as well as increased incidence of depressive symptoms among patients at the end of 1 year.

Monitoring and Troubleshooting
While patients are on the mechanical ventilator, various parameters have to be monitored such as blood pressure, respiratory rate, heart rate, and end-tidal carbon dioxide. Depending on the mode of ventilation, the volume achieved, pressures, or flow has to be monitored, and a close note should be made of the ventilator waveforms. The alarms can help to identify the problems associated with MV and to troubleshoot them.

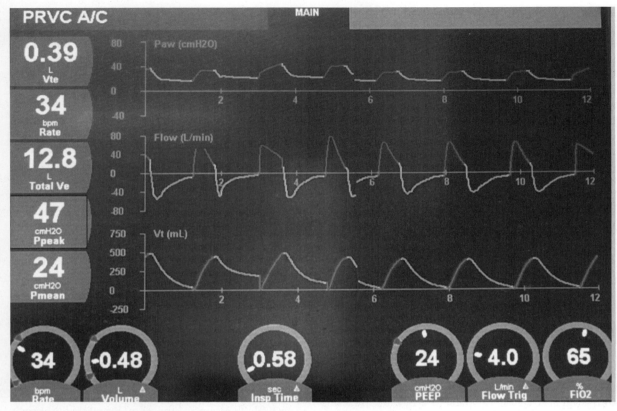

FIGURE 9-5. Parameter display on MV. (See color insert.)

One of the major problems encountered with MV is asynchrony between the vigorous spontaneous breaths by the patient and machine-delivered breaths. This results when there is increased respiratory drive and patients have a premature termination of the inspiratory flow and that, in turn, leads to insufficient ventilation.

This asynchrony can be mitigated by a couple of methods, including increasing the frequency of the breaths and

■ TABLE 9-6. Modes of Mechanical Ventilation			
Mode	**Trigger**	**Types of Breath**	**Dependent Variable**
Volume assist control	Time, flow, or pressure	Assisted or controlled	Pressure
Pressure assist control	Time, flow, or pressure	Assisted or controlled	Tidal volume
Pressure support ventilation	Flow or pressure	Supported	Tidal volume
SIMV (VC- or PC-IMV)	Time, flow, or pressure	Assisted or controlled	Minute ventilation
APRV (PC-IMV)	Time	Assisted or controlled	Tidal volume
PRVC (PC-CMV)	Time, flow, or pressure	Assisted or controlled	Minute ventilation
PAV (CSV)	Flow or pressure	Assisted	Pressure proportional to inspiratory effort
CPAP (CSV)	Flow or pressure	Assisted	

Abbreviations: APRV, airway pressure release ventilation; CMV, continuous mandatory ventilation; CPAP, continuous positive airway pressure; CSV, continuous spontaneous ventilation; IMV, intermittent mandatory ventilation; PAV, proportional assist ventilation; PC, pressure control; PRVC, pressure-regulated volume control; SIMV, synchronized intermittent mandatory ventilation; VC, volume control.

increasing the inspiratory flow. Sometimes, it requires increasing sedation, and in rare cases, even neuromuscular blockade can be used.

Tracheostomy Collar

A tracheostomy collar is a frequently used device in patients being liberated from long-term ventilation or in patients with tracheostomies done emergently. It is a soft, flexible plastic mask that fits around the tracheostomy tube. It is used to administer humidified oxygen or humidified air to the patient. The tracheostomy collar is used as a form of unassisted ventilatory support. It has been found to have shorter median weaning times compared to pressure support ventilation in patients who have been under long-term ventilator support (>21 days).

Vest-Chest Physiotherapy or High-Frequency Chest Wall Oscillations

Vest-chest physiotherapy is an evolved form of mechanical percussion or clapping of the chest that was historically done to clear respiratory secretions.

Mechanism of Action

The high-frequency chest wall oscillations, with rapid chest wall compressions and rapid elastic recoil of the chest wall, generate short pulses of respiratory flow that are believed to create biphasic changes in the transrespiratory pressure forcing secretions into larger airways. Studies have demonstrated that vest-chest physiotherapy increases airway clearance as evidenced by the mucus volume measurements compared to no chest physiotherapy.

Equipment

Vest-chest physiotherapy consists of a vest that is inflatable with the help of hoses connected to a generator that inflates the vest with pulses of air. Although the exact physiologic mechanism of airway clearance is yet to be understood, it is hypothesized that vest-chest physiotherapy helps loosen the adherent biofilm-forming secretions in the airways and helps the patient to cough out the secretions.

Complications With Vest-Chest Physiotherapy

- Acute hypotension or hypoxemia during therapy
- Increased intracranial pressure
- Pulmonary hemorrhage
- Musculoskeletal or spinal pain and injury
- Acute bronchospasm

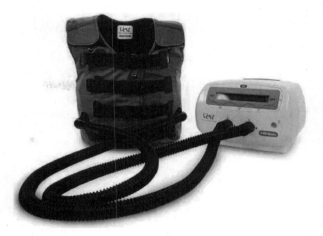

FIGURE 9-6. Chest vest equipment.

- Cardiac dysrhythmias
- Vomiting and aspiration

Monitoring and Troubleshooting

- The device manufacturer's instructions should be followed during the vest-chest physiotherapy. Ideally, the patient should be upright or in a sitting position during the therapy and should be concomitantly using bronchodilators.

■ **TABLE 9-7. Indications and Contraindications of Vest-Chest Physiotherapy**

Indications of vest-chest physiotherapy
Neuromuscular disorders: Motor neuron disease, cerebral palsy, muscular dystrophy and other myopathies, functional quadriplegia
Cystic fibrosis
Bronchiectasis
Cavitating lung disease
Atelectasis suspected or confirmed due to mucus plugging
Pneumonia in dependent lung regions
Pulmonary insufficiency following surgery or trauma

Contraindications of vest-chest physiotherapy
Bleeding diathesis, therapeutic anticoagulation
Active hemorrhage with hemodynamic instability
Unstable head or neck injury
Recent or active hemoptysis
Rib fractures, vertebral fractures
Elevated intracranial pressure
Empyema
Bronchopleural fistula
Pulmonary edema due to congestive cardiac failure

■ TABLE 9-8. Summary of Respiratory Devices	
Devices	**Mechanism of Action**
Bilevel noninvasive ventilation	Improves the alveolar gas exchange, improves the alveolar ventilation, and prevents the closure of the upper airway
High-flow nasal cannula (HFNC)	Leads to carbon dioxide washout, reduces the anatomic dead space, and reduces the work of breathing; increases alveolar recruitment, reduces airflow resistance, enhances oxygenation
Mechanical ventilator (MV)	Increases the lung volume by preventing atelectasis, improves gas exchange by maintaining ventilation and oxygenation, and reduces the work of breathing
Tracheostomy collar	Used as a form of unassisted ventilator strategy
Vest-chest therapy	Is a mechanical percussion device that helps to clear respiratory secretions

- The procedure should be performed before meals or at least 1 hour after eating. The therapy is usually initiated at low pressures and oscillatory frequencies and up-titrated as per patient tolerance. Each session lasts for 20 to 30 minutes.
- The vest-chest therapy can be used over implantable pumps, invasive monitoring lines, ports, or feeding tubes with adequate padding of the site. The session needs to be terminated immediately if the patient develops worsening pain, hypoxia, hypotension, or active hemoptysis.

■ FUTURE DIRECTIONS

- Efforts are ongoing to devise a ventilator that safely interacts with lung parenchyma to reduce ventilator-associated lung injury.
- Artificial intelligence–mediated algorithms have been proposed that can analyze respiratory/clinical status and guide the physician to troubleshoot issues.
- Regional ventilation based on lung mechanics is another area of interests and may improve respiratory care in the future.

REFERENCES

1. Nava S, Hill N. Non-invasive ventilation in acute respiratory failure. *Lancet.* 2009;374(9685):250-259.
2. Ram FS, Lightowler JV, Wedzicha JA. Non-invasive positive pressure ventilation for treatment of respiratory failure due to exacerbations of chronic obstructive pulmonary disease. *Cochrane Database Syst Rev.* 2003;1:CD004104. Update in: *Cochrane Database Syst Rev.* 2004;1:CD004104.
3. Rochwerg B, Brochard L, Elliott MW, et al. Official ERS/ATS clinical practice guidelines: noninvasive ventilation for acute respiratory failure. *Eur Respir J.* 2017;50(2):1602426.

Abbreviations

BiPAP: Bilevel positive airway pressure
CI: Confidence interval
CPAP: Continuous positive airway pressure, with no inspiratory assistance above the set pressure level
HFNC: High-flow nasal cannula
ICU: Intensive care unit
MV: Mechanical ventilation
NIV: Noninvasive ventilation
PEEP: Positive end-expiratory pressure
ROX: Respiratory rate oxygenation
RR: Relative risk

CHAPTER 10

Remote Monitoring Devices and General Concepts of Echocardiography

- *Vibha Hayagreev, MD; Sai Vishnuvardhan Allu, MD; Emamuzo Obaro Otobo, MD*

■ CASE PRESENTATION

A 40-year-old man presented with past medical history of New York Heart Association (NYHA) class III heart failure with ejection fraction of 35%, atrial fibrillation, status post cardioversion 2 times, and nonischemic cardiomyopathy. Other comorbid conditions include diabetes mellitus, hyperlipidemia, and hypertension. The patient presented to the hospital with worsening dyspnea, decreased exercise tolerance, and pedal edema for 1 week. During the previous year, he had 5 hospitalizations for acute decompensated heart failure and continued to struggle with volume management on an outpatient basis.

The patient's home medications include amiodarone 200 mg once a day, carvedilol 25 mg 2 times a day, sacubitril/valsartan (Entresto) once a day, aspirin, atorvastatin 40 mg at bedtime, apixaban (Eliquis) 5 mg 2 times a day, and torsemide 40 mg 2 times a day.

On examination, blood pressure is 118/90 mmHg, heart rate is 78 bpm with an irregularly irregular rhythm with holosystolic murmur at apex, and there is positive jugular venous distention, crackles from base-midlung bilaterally, and bilateral pitting pedal edema.

Significant laboratory values included elevated pro-B-type natriuretic peptide to 30,000 ng/dL (baseline 20,000-25,000) and creatinine of 1.8 mg/dL (baseline 1.4). Ultrasound of bilateral lower extremities was negative for deep vein thrombosis but positive for subcutaneous edema.

This patient was referred to heart failure management with CardioMEMS implantation.

■ KEY POINTS

- Several studies have shown that patients with NYHA class III heart failure, managed with an implantable hemodynamic monitoring system, had significant reduction in hospitalization regardless of their ejection fraction. This additional information about pulmonary artery pressure in addition to clinical findings facilitates efficient management.
- Remote heart rate monitoring devices have been used for arrhythmia detection, especially in diagnosis of atrial fibrillation in stoke patients.

■ INTRODUCTION

The global reach of modern technology, coupled with significant advances in computational power, marks a milestone of newfound potential in the development of digital health systems.

Although telemedicine is not a new concept, the widespread emergence of remote health monitoring initiatives across the United States has sparked fresh enthusiasm for the potential of next-generation digital tools to bridge pervasive gaps in the accessibility, affordability, and quality of healthcare.

For individuals managing chronic medical conditions, remote monitoring initiatives could create enabling environments of supported self-management and better personalized treatment plans. Remote sensor technologies allow healthcare to continue beyond the traditional clinical setting.

Such devices can be handheld, implanted, worn, or placed in the surrounding environment to capture health data and then electronically transmit that information back to healthcare providers for assessment. Several remote monitoring devices are described in Table 10-1. For the sake of convenience, only pertinent ones will be discussed in detail.

■ CARDIOMEMS

Introduction

The most updated and current clinical trials in management of heart failure have shown that a wireless implantable hemodynamic monitoring system such as CardioMEMS significantly decreases the rate of recurrent hospitalizations. This advanced technology is currently a class IIb indication in patients with New York Heart Association (NYHA) class III symptoms and a history of hospitalization in the past year regardless of ejection fraction.

Mechanism of Action

CardioMEMS is a small implantable pressure sensor with a micro-electromechanical system and piezoelectrical membrane placed in the left pulmonary artery to detect pulmonary artery pressures and transmit remotely to

■ TABLE 10-1. Types of Remote Devices

CardioMEMS
Implantable loop recorder (discussed in arrhythmia chapter)
Cardiac implantable electronic device remote monitoring
Ambulatory blood pressure monitoring
Heart rate monitors

the clinician. This can help guide the physician to titrate the diuretics in heart failure patients and hence reduces adverse outcomes.

Indications

The main goals of pressure-guided therapy are to:

- Understand the most current volume status of the patient on a day-to-day basis and thus predict the upcoming decompensation
- Optimize patients' current medical therapy and thus reduce recurrent hospital admissions

In addition, CardioMEMS can be used during acute decompensation events as a critical tool to guide intrahospital interventions such as inotrope infusion or left ventricular (LV) assist device monitoring, with the goal of securing an optimal volume status.

Contraindications

CardioMEMS should not be placed in patients with the following conditions:

- Coagulopathy
- Active infection
- Unable to take dual antiplatelet therapy for 1 month after procedure
- Recurrent pulmonary embolism/deep vein thrombosis
- Mechanical right-sided valves
- Noncompliance or unable to use the technology

Equipment

CardioMEMS consists of the following:

- Wireless pressure sensor
- Patient electronic system
- Patient database software

Procedure

CardioMEMS implantation is a very-low-risk procedure that includes percutaneous delivery of a pressure sensor into the branch of left pulmonary artery accessed via the femoral vein. It can facilitate constant telemetric pressure monitoring via a receiver.

Troubleshooting

In case of any changes in waveforms, dislodgement or malposition should be considered, and based on suspicion, the device should be recalibrated.

Table 10-2 summarizes the management and troubleshooting of data received from CardioMEMS.

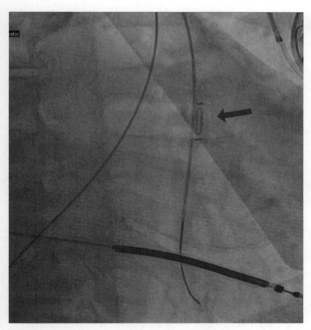

FIGURE 10-1. Fluoroscopy image showing CardioMEMS device.

Complications

- Access site complications include bleeding, vessel injury, and perforation.
- The most common adverse event is hemoptysis or pulmonary injury, with an overall complication rate of 2%.

TABLE 10-2. Troubleshooting CardioMEMS Data		
Data	**Intervention**	**Follow-Up**
Low PA pressure	Lower or hold diuretics, encourage hydration	Reevaluate in 48 hours
Normal PA pressure	No adjustment needed	Weekly or biweekly follow-up
Elevated PA pressure	Increase diuretic dose	Reevaluate in 48 hours

Abbreviation: PA, pulmonary artery.

- Sensor failure, migration, or malfunction can occur, requiring recalibrations and reimplantation.

■ HEART RATE MONITORS/ REMOTE CARDIAC MONITORING

Remote heart rate monitoring can be used to detect arrhythmia in high-risk patients such as patients with heart failure, myocardial infraction, stroke, or syncope. Heart rate monitors can be handheld, a patch, or app based. These monitors can be used in the hospital or at home for several days, and the information can be reviewed by the healthcare professional.

Mechanism of Action

A heart rate monitor consists of a fiber optic sensor that detects the heart rate either by electoral conduction,

Taken on: 03-16-2023, 11:18 AM

	PA Systolic	PA Mean	PA Diastolic	Heart Rate
Sensor:	71 mmHg	45 mmHg	29 mmHg	70 bpm
Reference:	—	45 mmHg	—	

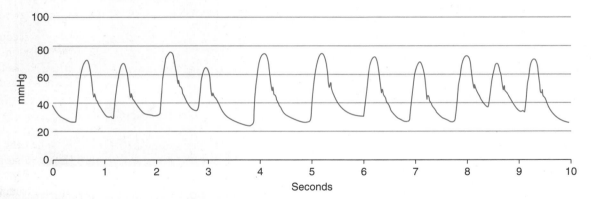

FIGURE 10-2. Tracing of CardioMEMS device. PA, pulmonary artery.

■ TABLE 10-3. Types of Arrhythmia Monitors		
Type	**Significance**	**Limitations**
Holter monitor	Continuous electrocardiogram recording, wearable	Monitoring for a few weeks
Event monitor	Symptom-based trigger for longer duration, wearable	Monitoring for 30 days, does not provide burden of arrhythmia
Patch monitor	Adhesive wearable, more portable than event monitor	Monitoring for 2 weeks
New-generation devices (smart phones and watches)	Continuous app-based monitoring	Artifacts and limited interpretation
Cardiac implantable electronic device remote cardiac monitor	Implantable device-based monitoring for continuous event detection, heart failure fluid management	Chances of artifacts, patient is out of range

electromagnetic impedance, infrared thermal imaging, or light intensity sensing. This information is recorded and delivered to a software-based data system for review.

Equipment

There are several types of monitors, as outlined in Table 10-3 and shown in Figure 10-3.

Indications and Contraindications

- A heart rate monitor is used for symptoms such as palpitation, dizziness, and syncope for detection of arrhythmia.
- It can be used after myocardial infraction for detection of malignant arrhythmia.
- It can be used in cases of stroke when atrial fibrillation/flutter is suspected.
- It can be used to detect efficacy and safety of antiarrhythmia therapy.
- It can be used to stratify risk of sudden cardiac death.
- The device should not be used in patients with no symptoms or when information cannot be interpreted by an expert, such as app-based events.

Complications and Troubleshooting

- To prevent artifacts, electrodes should be appropriately attached, and excessive moisture can affect the detection of events.
- Skin irritation or allergic reaction can occur due to electrodes.
- High magnetic areas should be avoided when the cardiac monitor is attached.

Future Directions

Artificial intelligence will increasingly be implemented to improvise diagnostics in remote monitoring devices

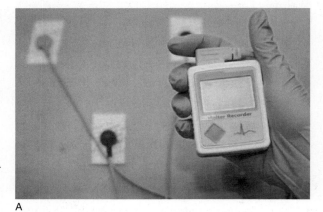

A

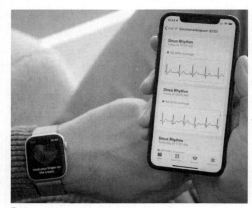

B

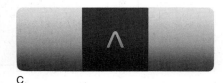

C

FIGURE 10-3. A-C. Various types of heart rate monitors. (See color insert.)

that will ultimately improve the quality of care and clinical outcomes.

BASICS OF ECHOCARDIOGRAPHY

Introduction

Echocardiography is imaging of the heart using standard ultrasound or Doppler ultrasound. The visual image formed using this technique is called an echocardiogram. In the current era of critical care, the diagnosis, treatment, and follow-up of patients with any suspected or established heart disorders require echocardiography. Echocardiography is one of the most frequently used diagnostic imaging techniques in cardiovascular conditions. It can provide a variety of useful information, from anatomy to hemodynamic assessment such as the size and shape of the heart (quantification of internal chamber size), pumping ability, location and severity of any tissue damage, and evaluation of the valves. Hemodynamic assessments of the heart, such as the computation of stroke volume, cardiac output, ejection fraction, and diastolic function, can also be made by clinicians using echocardiography.

Mechanism of Echocardiography

Echocardiography uses high-frequency sound waves (also called ultrasound) to image the heart. Standard echocardiography systems consist of the following:

- Transducer: The transducer sends the sound waves through the probe. The sound waves bounce off of the heart and return to the transducer as echoes.
- Computerized system: The computerized system processes and converts the echoes into images.
- Monitor: The images are displayed on a television monitor to produce pictures of the heart.

The 2 main types of echocardiograms are transthoracic echocardiograms (TTEs) and transesophageal echocardiograms (TEEs).

TRANSTHORACIC ECHOCARDIOGRAM

TTE is the most commonly used cardiac imaging modality, is noninvasive, and is fully performed outside of the body. TTE is a clinical tool for assessing the anatomy and physiology of the heart. TTE can evaluate all 4 chambers and respective valves, with standard images. It can utilize 4 imaging windows with various modalities including Doppler, M mode, and tissue Doppler imaging to obtain

relevant clinical information. Additional structures such as the aorta, pericardium, pleural effusions, ascites, and inferior vena cava can also be seen on TTE.

Modes of Echocardiogram

A-Mode

Modern echocardiography does not use amplitude mode.

2-Dimensional in B-Mode

Brightness mode is frequently used in conjunction with 2-dimensional imaging in echocardiography.

M-Mode

This mode has specific applications and the advantage of having extremely high temporal fidelity (eg, determining LV size at end diastole).

Doppler

Color Doppler

Color Doppler displays the structures' Doppler shift as color. Red and blue are typically used to represent this, with red denoting movement toward the transducer and blue denoting movement away from the transducer. This can be used to visually demonstrate the direction of blood flow by demonstrating blood flow through the valves.

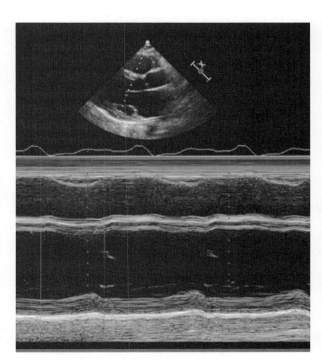

FIGURE 10-4. M-mode echocardiography.

Blood flow irregularities may be caused by valve stenosis and regurgitation. Blood flow in unusual places, such as with septal defects (atrial septal defect or ventricular septal defect), can also be seen with color Doppler.

Spectral Doppler

Both "continuous" and "pulse" waves can exhibit this, with the former displaying the spectrum along a particular line and the latter displaying inside a narrow window along that line. Both pulse wave and continuous wave are superior at displaying maximum velocities and flow across a limited volume, respectively.

Spectral Doppler is frequently used to quantify flow. By measuring the velocity time integral (VTI) of the aortic valve and LV outflow tract, for instance, one can estimate the area of the aortic valve using the continuity equation.

Indications and Contraindications

TTE can be used for the following conditions as outlined by appropriate use criteria:

- Initial evaluation when symptoms or signs suggest heart disease
- In the setting of newly diagnosed arrhythmia with or without symptoms such as ventricular tachycardia, nonsustained ventricular tachycardia, new-onset atrial fibrillation, or new left bundle branch block
- Assessment of syncope or near-syncope, hemodynamic instability, or volume
- Newly diagnosed hypertensive heart disease, LV dysfunction, complications of myocardial infraction, wall motion abnormality, evaluation of dyspnea, and pulmonary hypertension
- Evaluation of valvular heart disease, either native or prosthetic valve pathology, such as vegetation, tumor, or thrombus
- Assessment of pericardial disease, tumors, post-transplantation surveillance, and suspected aortic syndromes
- Part of preprocedure workup for structural heart procedure for accurate measurements such as patent foramen ovale closure or percutaneous valve placement

TTE should not be performed in asymptomatic patients with no cardiac risk factors.

Procedure

A complete echocardiogram is performed in multiple windows and axes. The function is assessed in multiple views.

Each view has a specific significance to analyze a specific cardiac structure.

Axes

The long axis and short axis are the 2 major axes of the heart.

- The long axis is a hypothetical line that passes through the middle of the tricuspid or mitral valve, depending on the reference ventricle.
- The heart's cross-section can be seen on the short axis, which is parallel to the long axis. For each valve, axes are also defined, with the long axis being the direction of blood flow and the short axis being the direction perpendicular to the flow.

Windows

- Parasternal: Adjacent to sternum. This implies without qualification that the right parasternal views but the left side of the heart can be sought.
- Apical: Located at the heart's peak.
- Subcostal: Near the top of the abdomen, beneath the sternum.
- Suprasternal: Near the base of the neck, above the sternum.

Views

Parasternal Long Axis View

This image, which shows the heart in its long axis, is obtained to the left of the sternum. The left atrium, right ventricular outflow tract, base of the LV, and mitral and aortic valves can all be seen in this image. The right ventricular inflow tract and tricuspid valve can be seen by angling this image, while the pulmonary valve can be seen by angling the opposite way.

The long-axis cross-section of the mitral and aortic valves can be seen in this view. In this view, it is also possible to see the typical "hockey stick" shape of rheumatic mitral stenosis. However, the angle of the probe with these valves may cause valve dysfunction to be underappreciated.

Visible structures include the following:

- Anterior septal and inferior lateral walls of the LV
- Left atrium
- Mitral valve in long axis with chordae
- Aortic valve in long axis
- Tricuspid valve in long axis (angulated) and right ventricular inflow tract
- Pulmonary valve in long axis (angulated) and right ventricular outflow tract

Measurements in this view can be used to assess the heart:

- LV size and wall thickness
- Left atrial linear dimension (as opposed to area)
- LV outflow tract diameter (used to calculate aortic valve area by the continuity equation)
- Aortic annulus, sinus of Valsalva, and aortic root sizes
- Color Doppler of all 4 valves
- Spectral Doppler of tricuspid and pulmonary valves

Parasternal Short Axis View

The probe is rotated 90 degrees to obtain the parasternal short axis view, which is obtained through the same window as the parasternal long axis view. The right ventricular input and outflow pathways, as well as the tricuspid valve, are visible in this view, together with the aortic valve in cross-section. In this view, the pulmonary valve is not discernible. The left and right atria are both discernible.

The following can be seen in this view:

- Short axis aortic valve
- Dysfunction of the aortic valve and aortic stenosis
- Long axis tricuspid valve
- Lung valve in the long axis
- Inflow and outflow passages and right ventricle
- Short axis LV
- LV outflow tract when one is nearer to the base
- The mitral valve leaflets' short axis movement at the base level
- Papillary muscles at the mid-LV level

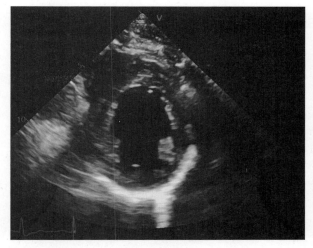

FIGURE 10-6. Parasternal short axis view.

In this view, the heart can be measured using the following methods:

- Area of the aortic valve using planimetry
- Each of the 4 valves using color Doppler
- Tricuspid and pulmonary valves using spectral Doppler

Apical 4-Chamber View

This view is achieved by standing at the top of the heart and gazing down toward the heart's base, which is where the valves are located. The tricuspid valve, mitral valve, and all 4 chambers are all visible in this image. This view, which depicts the right ventricle from base to apex, can be used to determine the right ventricle's systolic function. Additionally, tricuspid annular plane systolic excursion can be measured in this view using M-mode through the lateral tricuspid annulus.

The structures visible in this view include the following:

- Inferior septum and anterior lateral segments of the LV
- Right ventricle
- Left atrium
- Right atrium
- Mitral valve
- Tricuspid valve

Measurements in this view can be used to assess the following:

- RV size and function
- Left atrial size
- Right atrial size

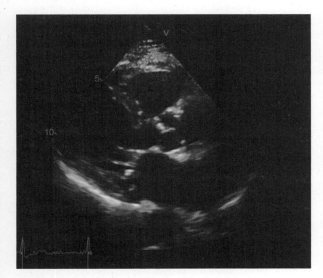

FIGURE 10-5. Parasternal long axis image.

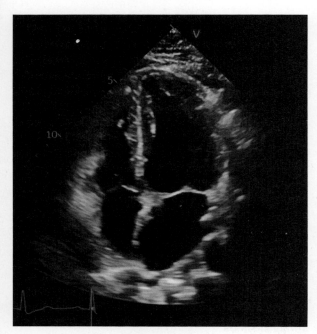

FIGURE 10-7. Apical 4-chamber view.

- Mitral valve flow, which best seen in this view and has the best angle with probe to estimate flows
- Tricuspid valve flow
- Tissue Doppler at the mitral valve annulus (septum and lateral wall) for diastolic function
- Agitated saline bubble study for right-to-left shunting (patent foramen ovale, atrial septal defect, ventricular septal defect)
- With contrast, apical and mural LV thrombi

Apical 3-Chamber View

Structures seen in the view include the following:

- Aortic valve
- Mitral valve
- LV
- Left atrium

Measurements in this view can be used to assess the following:

- LV outflow tract volume to be used in conjunction with aortic valve VTI for aortic valve area and stenosis
- Mitral valve flow

Apical 2-Chamber View

Structures seen in this view include the following:

- Anterior and inferior segments of the LV
- Mitral valve in long axis
- Left atrium

Measurements in this view can be used to assess the following:

- Mitral valve flow
- Spectral Doppler of the mitral valve

Subcostal View

This view is taken near the top of the abdomen and below the sternum. The intersection of the right atrium and inferior vena cava is most clearly visible in this image. Some people may be able to see similar views of the parasternal brief views and the apical 4 chambers through this window. These typical views may be available in some patients through a subcostal window rather than a parasternal or apical window due to various conditions such as chest wall injuries, open wounds, or inadequate acoustic windows. The inferior vena cava can only be seen through the subcostal window, and its size and collapsibility provide information that can be used to estimate the central venous pressure.

Suprasternal View

This view is obtained above the sternum in the suprasternal notch. In this view, the aortic arch and portion of the descending aorta can be seen. Color and spectral Doppler

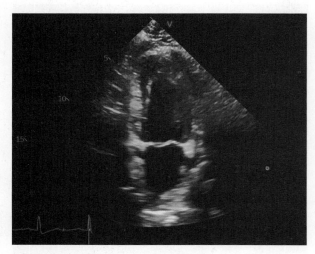

FIGURE 10-8. Apical 2-chamber view.

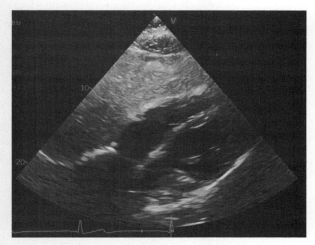

FIGURE 10-9. Subcostal view.

through the descending aorta can show signs of coarctation of the aorta.

■ TRANSESOPHAGEAL ECHOCARDIOGRAPHY

TEE is a semi-invasive procedure because it requires a probe to enter the body but does not involve any surgical (invasive) cutting. To reduce the gag reflex and improve the patient's discomfort, light to moderate sedation is administered before the probe is inserted. Typically, the

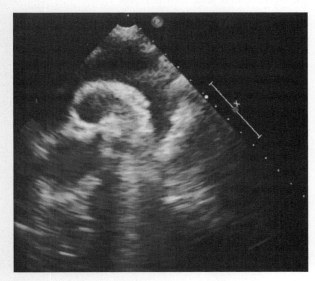

FIGURE 10-10. Suprasternal view.

back of the throat is treated with a local anesthetic spray (eg, lidocaine, benzocaine, or xylocaine) or the esophagus with a jelly or lubricant anesthetic. Because the procedure would be significantly diminished by the patient moving around, coughing, vomiting, and biting the probe, sedation and anesthesia are necessary to make the procedure comfortable and safe.

The probe is inserted through the mouth and into the esophagus after the patient has received sufficient sedative and anesthesia. The procedure's routine is exceedingly erratic after this point. The structures of great interest could be seen first because the study could end at any time (eg, respiratory compromise, hypotension, or intolerance to the probe). For instance, the mitral valve may be thoroughly examined initially if the TEE is required to check for mitral regurgitation. The probe is taken out at the end of the procedure, and the patient is watched to make sure they awake.

Indications and Contraindications

TEE can be used in the following conditions:

- For evaluation of left and right ventricle for hemodynamic assessment
- Assessment of valvular morphology and function, including thrombus, vegetation, and tumor evaluation
- Assessment of patients with suspected prosthetic valve dysfunction
- Evaluation of the left atrium and right atrium including appendage anatomy, including pulmonary vein size and inflow pattern, vena cava, and interatrial septum

Absolute contraindications include perforated viscus/esophagus and active upper gastrointestinal tract bleeding. Relative contraindications include esophageal varices, active peptic ulcer disease or a diagnosis of active esophagitis, recent upper gastrointestinal tract bleeding, Barrett esophagus, and restriction of neck mobility. Other contraindications include major risks, such as death, major bleeding, and esophageal and gastric perforation requiring open surgical repair, and minor risks, such as tracheal intubation, dysphagia, dental and lip injury, hoarseness, and minor bleeding.

Equipment

Probe

Most TEE probes contain a 2-dimensional ultrasound crystal. This permits rotation of the 2-dimensional echo

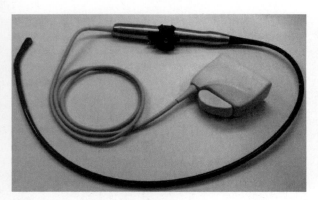

FIGURE 10-11. TEE probe.

plane without physical movement of the probe. In many cases, the probes have 1 or 2 degrees of freedom.

- The crystal may be pointed upward or downward by flexion or retroflexion, respectively.
- The probe tilts left and right due to left and right flexion.
- The dials on the probe's handle are often used to alter these 2 degrees. Axial rotation of the probe (clockwise or counterclockwise) constitutes a third degree of freedom and exists irrespective of the other two. The probe's translation along its axis to allow passage via the mouth, esophagus, and stomach is the fourth degree of translation.
- The combination of these 4 degrees of freedom permits 2-dimensional, color, and Doppler echocardiography of practically every structure in the heart.

Positions

TTE is used far more frequently than TEE because TEE can only visualize the heart through the windows that are available through the chest wall.

Mid-esophageal

The left atrium is positioned posterior to the mid-esophageal view, which at an angle of 0 degrees allows for a long-axis 4-chamber view. With a modest retroflexion of the probe, the long-axis 4-chamber view can be obtained at 0 degrees. To view the right heart and tricuspid valve, however, a small rotation and insertion may be required.

The aortic valve's short axis view is visible at a 45-degree angle. The right atrium, tricuspid valve, right ventricle, and pulmonary valve can all be seen in one view from this angle thanks to a short axis view of the right ventricle. When the probe is turned 90 degrees clockwise,

the bicaval view is obtained, allowing one to see the right atrium as well as the inferior and superior vena cava. The long axis image of the aortic valve can be seen at 135 degrees.

Transgastric

Pushing the TEE probe past the gastroesophageal junction into the stomach and flexing the probe (pointing it toward the superior) yields a short axis view of the heart. At 0 degrees, the short axis of the LV can be obtained to see wall motion in the basal, mid, and distal sections.

If the probe is rotated clockwise, then the right heart and tricuspid valve can be visualized. The transgastric position is best used to quantify the aortic valve with pulse and continuous wave Doppler, as this is the best view to be coaxial with the valve.

Upper Esophagus

The aortic arch can be seen when the TEE probe is pulled back further into the esophagus. The probe is often turned to reveal the descending aorta in the mid-esophageal view. The aorta and any atheromatous plaques inside can be seen by pulling back the probe. Aorta size measurements on the descending axis are possible at 0 degrees. The aortic arch will finally be reached with further withdrawal, and rotation in a clockwise direction will reveal the arch. Aortic coarctation can be seen by continuously imagining the aorta up to the level of the arch.

Complications and Limitations

Complications of TEE are listed in Table 10-4.

TEE has several limitations that need to be considered alongside its significant advantages. Patients undergoing TEE must comply with the NPO (nothing by mouth) recommendations, which often involve abstaining from eating or drinking for 8 hours before the procedure. Performing a TEE requires a team of medical professionals, including a doctor, an anesthesiologist, a nurse responsible for administering anesthesia, and a sonographer.

Compared to TTE, TEE typically takes longer to complete. Successful TEE procedures may necessitate the administration of general anesthesia, which can cause discomfort for the patient. The technical complexity of TEE is higher as it requires anesthesia and skilled execution to ensure accuracy and safety.

TEE is limited by the specific anatomy of each patient. For example, the risk associated with TEE can significantly increase if the patient has esophageal varices, esophageal stricture, Barrett esophagus, or other esophageal or

■ TABLE 10-4. TEE Complications

Gastrointestinal	Dental injury
	Pharyngeal injury
	Jaw subluxation
	Esophageal tear/perforation
	Bleeding
	Unsuccessful intubation
Respiratory	Hypoxia
	Bronchospasm
	Aspiration
	Supraglottic hematoma
Cardiovascular	Vasovagal reaction
	Malignant hypertension
	Heart block, tachy-/
	bradyarrhythmia
Infection	Probe contamination
Medication related	Methemoglobinemia
	Excessive sedation
	Seizure

stomach conditions. In such cases, an initial esophago-gastroduodenoscopy might be necessary to assess the anatomy and ensure safety, which may subject the patient to an additional procedure. Anatomic considerations can introduce an unacceptable level of risk.

Whereas TTE provides numerous measurements to aid in disease diagnosis and grading, TEE parameters are not as clearly established. Consequently, there are fewer widely recognized criteria, such as left atrial enlargement, for TEE analysis.

Troubleshooting

The range of an ultrasound machine's life span is influenced by its usage and the implementation of preventative maintenance measures. Approximately two-thirds of ultrasound machine failures can be attributed to software corruption and ultrasound transducer problems. The remaining troubleshooting primarily revolves around probe issues.

Software problems typically arise from improper machine shutdown procedures. Many instances involve abruptly cutting off the main power source instead of allowing the machine to shut down properly, resulting in abnormal software behavior and potential corruption. Ensuring a correct shutdown process is crucial to minimize the occurrence of such mishaps.

Hardware failures can be categorized into core hardware and input hardware issues. Input hardware failures encompass problems with barcode scanners, keyboards, cases, and other sensing equipment. Core hardware

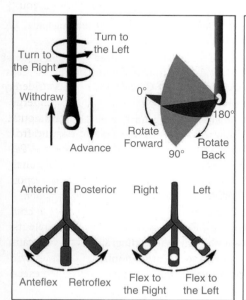
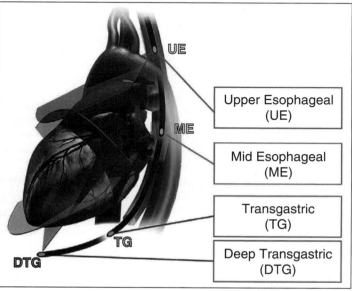

FIGURE 10-12. Views and position of TEE probe. (Reproduced with permission from Hahn RT, Abraham T, Adams MS, Bruce CJ, Glas KE, Lang RM, Reeves ST, Shanewise JS, Siu SC, Stewart W, Picard MH. Guidelines for performing a comprehensive transesophageal echocardiographic examination: recommendations from the American Society of Echocardiography and the Society of Cardiovascular Anesthesiologists. *J Am Soc Echocardiogr.* 2013;26(9):921-64.)

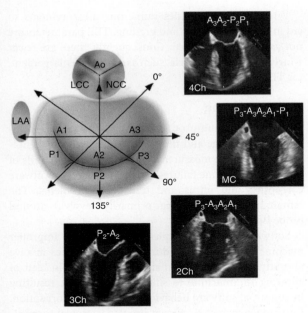

FIGURE 10-13. Views of TEE. Ao aorta; LAA, left atrial appendage; LCC, left coronary cusp; NCC, noncoronary cusp. (See color insert.) (Reproduced with permission from Hahn RT, Abraham T, Adams MS, Bruce CJ, Glas KE, Lang RM, Reeves ST, Shanewise JS, Siu SC, Stewart W, Picard MH. Guidelines for performing a comprehensive transesophageal echocardiographic examination: recommendations from the American Society of Echocardiography and the Society of Cardiovascular Anesthesiologists. *J Am Soc Echocardiogr.* 2013;26(9):921-64.)

failures involve the central computer processing units, batteries, and cables. While hardware failures are less common, they often necessitate component replacement when they occur.

Common problems encountered with ultrasound machines include the following:

1. Hardware issues
   - Failure of sensing equipment
   - Malfunctioning keyboard
   - Printer failure
   - Monitor malfunction
   - Processor failure
   - Storage failure

2. Probe/transducer issues
   - Compatibility issues between the probe and cable
   - Connectivity issues with the probe cable
   - Noise and vibration during operation
   - Electrical interference affecting image quality
   - Damaged or broken pins in the connector
   - Broken cables
   - Physical damage or breakage of the probe
   - Poor-quality image output
   - Tears on the sheath
   - Crystal damage
   - Connector issues
   - Cracked or air bubbles on the lens

3. Software issues
   - Virus/malware
   - Outdated version
   - Software corruption
   - Improper shutdown

Future Directions

Further advances in 3-dimensional echocardiography and strain imaging are ongoing to analyze cardiac mechanics and implement them into clinical practice.

SUGGESTED READINGS

Lang RM, Goldstein SA, Kronzon I, et al, eds. *ASE's Comprehensive Echocardiography.* 3rd ed. Philadelphia, PA: Elsevier; 2021.

Singh R, Scarfone S, Zughaib M. Wedged sensor in distress? Lessons learned from troubleshooting dampened transmitted PA waveforms of CardioMEMS device. *Case Rep Cardiol.* 2020;2020:3856940.

Tschöpe C, Alogna A, Spillmann F, et al. The CardioMEMS system in the clinical management of end-stage heart failure patients: three case reports. *BMC Cardiovasc Disord.* 2018;18(1):155.

Abbreviations

LV: Left ventricle
NYHA: New York Heart Association
TEE: Transesophageal echocardiography
TTE: Transthoracic echocardiography
VTI: Velocity time integral

CHAPTER 11

Lines and Catheters

• Sarthak Kulshreshtha, MD; Muhammad Saad, MD

■ CASE PRESENTATION

A 71-year-old woman with a past medical history of hypertension, morbid obesity (body mass index 41 kg/m²), diabetes mellitus, chronic obstructive pulmonary disease (COPD), stage 3 chronic kidney disease, advanced longstanding peripartum cardiomyopathy, and left ventricular ejection fraction 25% status post cardiac resynchronization therapy with defibrillator presented to the emergency department with worsening dyspnea on exertion and lower extremity swelling. She was started on intravenous (IV) furosemide infusion, and a repeat echocardiogram showed a left ventricular ejection fraction of less than 20% and a left ventricular outflow tract velocity time integral of 9 cm. She was started on IV milrinone 0.375 µg/kg/min infusion after frequent central venous oxygen saturation ($ScvO_2$) via a central venous catheter (CVC). She was in stage D heart failure with multiple relative contraindications for a heart transplant and advanced heart failure therapies, including age (71 years of age), renal failure (creatinine 2.5 mg/dL), obesity, moderate COPD, high panel-reactive antibody, and frailty. After 6 days of hospitalization, she was found to be euvolemic on the examination. Her central venous pressure was 9 mmHg, $ScvO_2$ was 68% with calculated Fick cardiac output of 5.2 L/min, and cardiac index was 2.6 L/min/m². In this case, CVC helps assess central venous pressure and $ScvO_2$ and estimate Fick cardiac output and cardiac index.

■ KEY POINTS

- Vascular catheters are essential tools in the management of critically ill cardiac patients, allowing clinicians to administer treatment, monitor vital signs, and obtain diagnostic information in real time.
- Antibiotic-impregnated catheters have recently been introduced to prevent risk of catheter-associated bloodstream infection.

■ INTRODUCTION

In managing patients in the cardiac care unit, various devices are used to manage patients optimally. These devices serve various purposes, including interventional, diagnostic, and therapeutic. These devices are crucial in the management of critically sick patients and have evolved over the years to improve the prognosis and offer better management options to medical staff all over the world.

This chapter provides an overview of various miscellaneous devices used in cardiac critical care, including lines and catheters. These devices monitor and support critically ill cardiac patients and provide them with the necessary care and treatment. This chapter will cover the importance of different types of lines and catheters, such as central lines, arterial lines, urinary catheters, vascular catheters, dialysis catheters, pleural drains, pericardial drains, and others commonly used in cardiac critical care (Table 11-1). This chapter will also cover some devices under development, providing an update on current research and prospects. Through this chapter, the readers will gain an understanding of the various lines and catheters used in cardiac critical care and the role they play in the management and treatment of critically ill cardiac patients.

■ TABLE 11-1. Types of Lines and Catheters			
Vascular Catheters	Drains	Nutritional Catheters	Output Catheter
Central venous lines	Pericardial	Gastrostomy tube	Urinary catheter
Arterial line	Pleural	Nasogastric tube	
Dialysis catheter		Total parenteral nutrition	

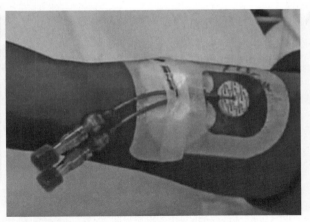

FIGURE 11-1. Peripherally inserted central catheter line. (See color insert.)

■ VASCULAR CATHETERS

Several types of vascular catheters are discussed in the following sections.

Central Lines

A vascular catheter is a thin, flexible tube that is inserted into a vein or artery for the purpose of administering fluids, medications, or nutrients or for measuring blood pressure. Vascular catheters can be used for many procedures, from routine blood draws to more complex medical treatments.

A central line is a type of catheter inserted into a large vein in the body, usually in the chest, neck, or groin.

Mechanism of Action

Central lines are used to administer medications, fluids, or nutrients, as well as to take blood samples. They are typically used in hospitals and other medical settings for patients who need frequent or prolonged treatment.

Indications and Contraindications

In cardiac critical care, vascular catheters play an important role in the management of critically ill patients. They can be used to deliver medications, fluids, and nutrition directly to the patient's circulatory system, which can help to maintain blood pressure, improve oxygenation, and support the function of vital organs such as the heart and kidneys.

There are no major contraindications for a arterial line except local infection or coagulopathy.

Equipment

There are different types of central lines, but they are broadly divided into 2 groups:

- A peripherally inserted central catheter is a long, thin tube inserted into a vein in the arm and passed through the chest to the heart.

- Tunneled catheters, or implantable venous access devices, are surgically implanted beneath the skin, typically in the chest, with a small bump (port) showing on the skin surface.

Complications and Troubleshooting

- There are various types of central lines, each with its own risks and benefits, depending on the patient's condition, the type and duration of treatment, and the level of invasiveness.
- Vascular catheters are generally considered safe. However, there are potential complications, such as infections, bleeding, thrombosis, or catheter occlusion. That is why it is important for the healthcare professional to carefully follow aseptic techniques and guidelines for catheter maintenance and care.
- These lines are typically used in critically ill patients who require frequent blood tests or need to receive a large amount of fluids, medications, or nutrition.
- Central lines allow easy access to the patient's central circulatory system, reducing the need for repeated needle sticks and increasing the precision of medical treatments.
- Chest X-ray is warranted after placing the central line to assess the location and rule out pneumothorax.

Arterial Lines

An arterial line, also known as an arterial catheter, is a thin, flexible tube inserted into an artery, typically in the wrist or the groin.

Mechanism of Action

Arterial line pressure measurement works on the principle of hydrostatic pressure using a column of fluid displayed electronically as a pressure waveform.

Equipment

- An arterial line kit contains sterile cleaning solution, arterial catheter, and suture material.
- Ultrasound machine for safe access.

Indications and Contraindications

- The purpose of an arterial line is to continuously monitor the patient's blood pressure, as well as to obtain frequent blood samples for testing.
- This type of line is mostly used in critically ill patients in the intensive care unit. They are used to measure the precise blood pressure and blood gas samples for monitoring acid-base balance, oxygenation, and other hemodynamic parameters.
- Arterial lines can also be used in the intensive care unit to monitor a patient's cardiac output. The information gathered from an arterial line can also be used to evaluate the patient's overall perfusion and tissue oxygenation, as well as to adjust treatments such as fluid and pressor therapy.
- Additionally, the arterial line is used to check the acid-base balance, which can be useful in treating the critically ill patient with respiratory problems such as acute respiratory distress syndrome or sepsis.
- There are no major contraindications for an arterial line except local infection or coagulopathy.

Complications and Troubleshooting

- Arterial lines have a higher risk of complications such as bleeding or artery damage at the insertion site, leading to fistula formation or dissection.
- Additionally, the procedure carries a slight risk of infection and occlusion of the line.
- Pressure should be measured at the phlebostatic angle with the transducer zeroed to avoid atmospheric pressure.
- Overdampening the waveform is seen as a sluggish waveform downstroke and may give underestimated pressures. Kinks, bubbles, and clots may cause it.
- Underdampening the waveform is seen as a spike and may give overestimated pressures. Tachycardia, catheter whip, or stiff catheter can lead to it.

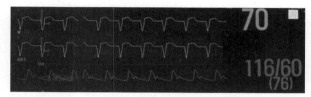

FIGURE 11-2. Arterial line waveform. (See color insert.)

- Excessive bleeding at insertion site may be secondary to coagulopathy and needs assessment by international normalized ratio and platelet check.

Dialysis Catheter

Dialysis catheters are commonly used in critically ill cardiac patients who have developed acute kidney injury (AKI) due to their cardiac condition. AKI can be caused by various factors, such as low blood pressure, decreased blood flow to the kidneys, or certain medications.

Dialysis catheters can be either tunneled or nontunneled. Tunneled catheters are inserted under the skin inside subcutaneous tissue to access the vein. Nontunneled catheters are placed over the skin.

Mechanism of Action

A dialysis catheter is a long (20 cm), 8- to 11-F tube inserted into a vein in the patient's neck or chest and then threaded through to the vena cava. The catheter has 2 separate lumens, or channels: one is used to remove blood from the body, and the other is used to return the blood to the patient's body after it has been treated.

Equipment

Similar to other central line placement, dialysis catheters use the same principle, with ultrasound guidance needed for safe vascular access.

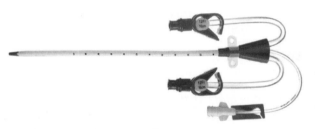

FIGURE 11-3. Dialysis catheter.

Indications and Contraindications

- In cardiac critical care, dialysis catheters can play an important role in the management of patients with renal failure, which is a common complication of cardiac disease.
- Dialysis catheters allow for the rapid and efficient removal of waste products and excess fluid from the blood, which can help to improve the patient's overall health and reduce the risk of further complications.
- There are no major contraindications for a dialysis catheter except local infection or coagulopathy.

Complications and Troubleshooting

- Inserting a dialysis catheter carries a risk of infection, bleeding, or damage to the vein or surrounding tissue.
- The catheter must be handled with care and with an aseptic technique to minimize the risk of complications.
- Failure of a dialysis catheter can be due to kinking, clot formation, or small vessel size.

■ URINARY CATHETER

A urinary catheter is a thin, flexible, silicone or latex tube that is inserted into the bladder through the urethra to drain urine. Urinary catheters play an important role in monitoring the fluid balance and kidney function of critically ill cardiac patients, providing clinicians with valuable information to help guide their treatment and care.

Mechanism of Action

There are different types of urinary catheters:

- External catheter: Attached to urethra to avoid incontinence
- Bladder catheter: Inserted directly into the bladder
- Urethral catheter: Inserted directly in the urethra

Indwelling urinary catheters are used in patients who have problems with urine output, such as urinary retention or incontinence.

Equipment

Equipment includes urinary catheter and sterile supplies.

Indications and Contraindications

In cardiac critical care, urinary catheters may be used to monitor urine output, providing important information about a patient's overall fluid balance and kidney

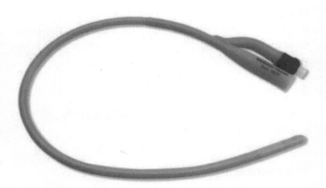

FIGURE 11-4. Foley catheter.

function. Urine output can indicate the patient's cardiac function, blood flow to the kidneys, and response to medical treatments.

Urine output is often closely monitored in critically ill cardiac patients in order to identify any signs of renal dysfunction or failure. A decrease in urine output can indicate a reduction in blood flow to the kidneys, which can be caused by low blood pressure or reduced cardiac output.

Additionally, the urinary catheter can be used to measure the pressure in the bladder; this is called a Foley catheter. It is done with a special type of catheter, with a balloon tip inflated once it is placed in the bladder. This method can be used to measure the pressure in the abdomen and to detect if there is a pressure increase called abdominal compartment syndrome.

There are no major contraindications, except local infection or trauma.

Complications and Troubleshooting

The use of a urinary catheter carries a risk of urinary tract infections as well as other complications such as bladder spasms, bleeding, and damage to the urethra. Careful hygiene and monitoring by healthcare professionals are essential to minimize these risks.

■ PLEURAL DRAIN

Pleural effusion is a common complication in patients with heart failure, lung infections, or cancer, among other conditions. The excess fluid or air can compress the lung and make breathing difficult, causing the patient to become short of breath and potentially leading to other complications such as atelectasis, pneumonia, or pleural infection. A pleural drain is used to remove fluid or air from the pleural cavity.

Mechanism of Action

- A pleural drain is a thin, flexible tube inserted through the chest wall and into the pleural space, which is the area between the lung and the chest wall.
- The purpose of a pleural drain is to remove excess fluid or air accumulated in the pleural space, a condition known as pleural effusion.

Equipment

- A pleural drain can be placed in several ways including the percutaneous approach or minimally invasive thoracotomy for video-assisted thoracoscopic surgery.
- Ultrasound guidance is required for safe access to pleural space.
- Repeat chest X-ray is required after placement to confirm location.

Indications and Contraindications

The procedure carries a small risk of infection, bleeding, and pneumothorax (air in the pleural space that can cause the lung to collapse). The duration of drainage depends on the condition of the patient; generally, it is removed when the fluid or air output decreases and the patient's symptoms improve.

In cardiac critical care, pleural drains may be used in patients who have developed pleural effusions as a complication of their cardiac condition, such as heart failure. In addition to heart failure, pleural effusions can also occur as a complication of certain lung infections, such as pneumonia, and certain types of cancer, especially lung cancer. In these cases, a pleural drain can be used to remove the excess fluid or air from the pleural space, which can help to alleviate shortness of breath and other symptoms and improve lung function.

A pleural drain can also be used to diagnose pleural effusions; often, the analysis of the pleural fluid can give the healthcare professional an idea of the underlying cause.

It's worth noting that pleural drain is considered an invasive procedure, and it's only done in critical care settings when noninvasive options such as diuretics and oxygen therapy are insufficient to manage the patient's condition.

Complications and Troubleshooting

- Major complications include pain, bleeding, leaking, and infection.
- Blocked or dislodged chest tubes should be removed.
- Clinical change warrants repeat chest X-ray.

■ PERICARDIAL DRAIN

Pericardial effusion is the accumulation of fluid in the pericardial sac. This condition can cause compression of the heart and lead to a decrease in cardiac output, which can result in symptoms such as chest pain, shortness of breath, and low blood pressure.

Mechanism of Action

A pericardial drain, also known as a pericardiocentesis, is a medical procedure in which a thin, flexible tube, called a pericardial catheter, is inserted through the chest and into the pericardial space, which is the area between the heart and the inner lining of the pericardium (the sac that surrounds the heart).

Equipment

- The procedure is typically done under local anesthesia and with the guidance of ultrasound or X-ray imaging.
- The pericardial catheter is inserted through the chest and into the pericardial space, where the excess fluid can be removed.

Indications and Contraindications

- Pericardial drains are typically used to treat conditions such as cardiac tamponade, a life-threatening condition caused by the accumulation of fluid in the pericardial sac that compresses the heart and impairs its ability to pump blood.
- Other conditions, such as pericarditis, which is an inflammation of the pericardium, and malignancy, are also common causes of pericardial effusion.

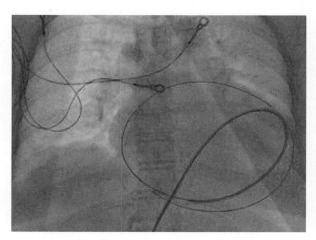

FIGURE 11-5. Pericardial catheter.

- Additionally, malignancies such as lung cancer and breast cancer can also cause pericardial effusion, a pericardial drain can be used to remove the fluid, relieve symptoms, and assist in the diagnosis and management of the malignancy.

Complications and Troubleshooting

- The procedure carries a small risk of bleeding, infection, pneumothorax, and arrhythmias.
- A blocked or dislodged pericardial drain should be removed.
- Clinical change warrants repeat transthoracic echocardiography.

■ NUTRITIONAL DEVICES

In cardiac critical care, nutritional devices can play an important role in the management of critically ill patients who are unable to take in enough nutrition through oral means or who have difficulty swallowing. These devices can give patients the nutrition they need to support their recovery and improve their overall health.

One nutrition device used in cardiac critical care is the enteral feeding tube. This tube is passed through the nose or mouth and into the stomach or small intestine to provide patients with enteral nutrition, a liquid or semi-liquid form of nutrition specially designed for patients who cannot eat or drink enough to meet their nutritional needs.

Another type of nutritional device is total parenteral nutrition (TPN), which provides complete nutrition to patients through intravenous fluids.

These devices can deliver nutrition to patients with recent surgery, such as open-heart surgery; those with severe neurologic conditions, such as stroke or brain injury; or patients with critical illnesses, such as sepsis or multiorgan failure. These devices can help prevent or treat malnutrition, which can be a complication of essential conditions and lead to poor wound healing, muscle weakness, and increased risk of infection.

It is essential to monitor the patient's response to the nutritional devices and to make sure that the devices are functioning properly and that they are being used correctly. It is also essential to monitor the patient's nutrient levels, electrolytes, and other values.

Gastrostomy Tubes

Patients in cardiac critical care who have had recent open-heart surgery, those with severe neurologic conditions

such as stroke or brain injury, or patients with a critical illness such as sepsis or multiorgan failure are at risk of developing malnutrition and complications related to poor nutrition. Gastrostomy tubes (G-tubes) can be used to provide these patients with the food and hydration they need to support their recovery and improve their overall health.

Mechanism of Action

In cardiac critical care, G-tubes can be inserted using less invasive endoscopic techniques, or they can be inserted surgically through a small incision in the abdominal wall. Once in place, the G-tube can provide the patient with enteral nutrition, a liquid or semi-liquid form of food specially designed for patients who cannot eat or drink enough to meet their nutritional needs.

Indications and Contraindications

- G-tubes can be used for patients who have difficulty swallowing or have conditions that make it difficult to absorb enough nutrients from oral food and fluids.
- G-tubes also can be used for other purposes such as medication administration, gastric decompression, and measurement of pH and gastrointestinal secretions.
- Sepsis, coagulopathy, severe ascites, and metastatic cancer in the peritoneum are general contraindications.

Complications and Troubleshooting

- It is important to note that using a G-tube carries a risk of infection, bleeding, blockage, and dislodgement.
- Granulation tissue can form due to leaking that may need barrier cream.
- Excessive leaking around tube should be assessed by checking balloon volume and checking the position of the G-tube.
- If the G-tube is clogged due to thick formula, try flushing with acidic fluid.
- It is essential for healthcare professionals to closely monitor and maintain the tube and ensure proper care and hygiene are in place to minimize the risk of complications.

Total Parenteral Nutrition in Cardiac Critical Care Unit

TPN provides complete nutrition to patients through intravenous (IV) fluids. In cardiac critical care, TPN may be used for patients who cannot take in enough food orally or through a G-tube, such as critically ill patients

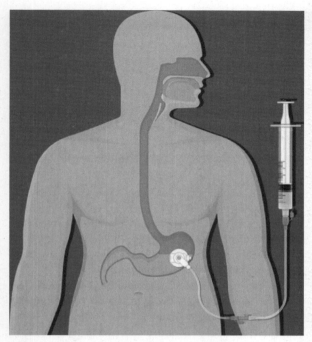

FIGURE 11-6. Gastrostomy tube (G-tube). (See color insert.) (Used with permission from Pepermpron/Shutterstock.)

who have had recent surgery, have severe neurologic conditions, or have a critical illness.

Mechanism of Action

TPN is a complex and specialized form of nutrition delivered directly into the bloodstream through a vein. It provides a balanced mixture of glucose, amino acids, fats, vitamins, and minerals that the body needs to function properly. TPN is typically administered through a central venous catheter, a long, thin tube inserted into a vein in the patient's neck or chest.

Components

- Lipid emulsions (25%-30%)
- Proteins (1.5 g/kg/day)
- Carbohydrates
- Electrolytes, multivitamins, and minerals

Indications and Contraindications

TPN can effectively provide critically ill patients with the nutrition they need to support their recovery and improve their overall health. It can help to prevent or treat malnutrition, which can be a complication of critical illness and can lead to poor wound healing, muscle weakness, and

increased risk of infection. TPN can also help to improve the patient's energy levels, reduce the risk of organ failure, and support the immune system. TPN should not be used to prolong life.

Complications

TPN is associated with certain risks and complications, including infection, bleeding, and emboli. It also requires close monitoring and management by healthcare professionals, including regular blood tests to check for signs of electrolyte imbalances or infection.

■ WOUND CARE IN CARDIAC CRITICAL CARE UNIT

A wound is any disruption in the skin and mucosal continuity. Leg ulcers and decubitus ulcers are common in cardiac critical care unit patients due to underlying medical conditions and bedridden state. Wound healing is the combination of improving underlying medical issues and nutritional status. It is important to understand the types of wounds and dressings to take care of critically ill patients. We will discuss pressure ulcers in this section.

For pressure ulcers, wound dressings are used to protect the wound and promote healing by providing a protective barrier between the wound and the surrounding skin, which can help to reduce the risk of infection and promote healing. They can also help to reduce pain, discomfort, and odor.

Management

All pressure or medical device–related wounds should be assessed for:

- Infection
- Moisture
- Sloughing, necrosis, or rolling edges

Wounds should be appropriately documented to guide type of dressing. Wounds should also be assessed for fistula formation.

There are different types of dressings in general use, including the following:

- Polyurethane foam dressing is an adsorbent padding used for stage I ulcers.
- Alginates can be applied on wet wounds and avoid excessive fluid and infection spread. They are used in infected wounds.
- Hydrogels are used for dry abrasions.

■ TABLE 11-2. Pressure Ulcer Wound Classifications

Partial Thickness	Full Thickness	Deep Tissue Injury	Unstageable Ulcer
Stage I Intact skin with nonblanchable redness	**Stage III** Subcutaneous tissue seen	Purple localized area of skin	Wound covered by eschar
Stage II Open shallow red wound with loss of dermis	**Stage IV** Exposed bone tendon or muscle		

- Hydrocolloid is an occlusive dressing to promote angiogenesis and granulation and to create a moist environment in dry wounds. Avoid if there is a risk of infection.
- Thin film is used for stage I or II ulcers to cover the wound.
- Cotton gauze is used to cover dressings, and wet to dry gauze can be used after debridement.
- Honey dressing is used for stage I or II ulcers.
- Silver dressing prevents epithelization and is used for infected wounds.
- Other options include negative-pressure wound therapy, phototherapy, and collagen-based dressings for advance nonhealing wounds.
- Eschar or unstageable wounds always require debridement for appropriate staging.

■ FUTURE DIRECTIONS

Several devices are currently under development for cardiac critical care management, including the following:

- Noninvasive hemodynamic monitoring devices measure vital signs such as blood pressure, heart rate, and cardiac output noninvasively, reducing the need for invasive catheterization and minimizing the risk of complications associated with invasive monitoring.
- Biomarker-based diagnostic devices aim to provide a rapid and accurate diagnosis of cardiac conditions by measuring biomarkers in blood or other bodily fluids, such as troponin, B-type natriuretic peptide, and pro-brain natriuretic peptide.

- Artificial intelligence–based devices provide real-time monitoring, analysis, and decision-making support for cardiac critical care management. These devices can help to identify patterns and predict outcomes, allowing healthcare providers to make more informed decisions and improve patient outcomes.
- Miniaturized mechanical circulatory support devices are designed to be less invasive and more portable than current devices for patients suffering from heart failure or cardiogenic shock and can be used for long-term support or as a bridge to transplant.

SUGGESTED READINGS

Farrell J, Gellens M. Ultrasound-guided cannulation versus the landmark-guided technique for acute haemodialysis access. *Nephrol Dial Transplant*. 1997;12:1234-1237.

Guyatt GH, Oxman AD, Vist GE, et al. GRADE: an emerging consensus on rating quality of evidence and strength of recommendations. *BMJ*. 2008;336:924-926.

Abbreviations

AKI: Acute kidney injury
COPD: Chronic obstructive pulmonary disease
CVC: Central venous catheter
G-tube: Gastrostomy tube
IV: Intravenous
$ScvO_2$: Central venous oxygen saturation
TPN: Total parenteral nutrition

Miscellaneous Devices

CHAPTER 12

• *Maheen Ali Khan, MD; Muhammad Hassan, MD; Muhammad Saad, MD*

■ CASE PRESENTATION

A 75-year-old woman was brought to the emergency department (ED) with altered mental status and lethargy by her son. The patient's son found her in bed with altered mental status for an unknown duration. At home, her vitals showed a pulse of 126 bpm, systolic blood pressure of 82/42 mmHg, and oxygen saturation of 89% on room air. Upon arrival at the ED, the patient received 1.5 L of normal saline and was placed on high-flow supplemental oxygen.

The patient's past medical history includes nonischemic cardiomyopathy (left ventricular ejection fraction of 30%), hypertension, paroxysmal atrial fibrillation, and recurrent urinary tract infections. She is currently taking metoprolol succinate, spironolactone, lisinopril, apixaban, and nitrofurantoin.

Upon examination in the ED, the patient remained minimally responsive, with a temperature of 39.3°C, heart rate of 114 bpm, blood pressure of 86/50 mmHg, and oxygen saturation of 88% on high-flow oxygen. Her physical examination revealed a normal S1 and S2, no S3 or S4, and a grade 2/6 mid-peaking systolic murmur at the left sternal border. Jugular veins were difficult to assess due to her body habitus, and lung fields were clear anteriorly. The patient's extremities were cool to the touch with sluggish capillary refill. The patient was intubated in the ED and received an additional 2 L of normal saline. She was subsequently transferred to the intensive care unit.

The patient's initial laboratory values (with normal reference values shown in parentheses) are as follows:
- Leukocyte count: 18,000/μL (4500-11,000/μL)
- Hemoglobin, blood: 11 g/dL (11.9-14.8 g/dL)
- Sodium: 128 mEq/L (135-145 mEq/L)
- Potassium: 3.7 mEq/L (3.5-5.0 mEq/L)
- Blood urea nitrogen: 44 mg/dL (7-18 mg/dL)
- Creatinine: 1.6 mg/dL (0.6-1.2 mg/dL)
- Lactate: 4.7 mmol/L (0.5-2.2 mmol/L)

A pulmonary artery (PA) catheter was placed, and findings were as follows:
- Right atrial pressure, mean: 8 mmHg (1-5 mmHg)
- Right ventricular pressure: 50/20 mmHg (15-30 mmHg/4-12 mmHg)
- PA pressure: 50/15 mmHg (mean 28 mmHg)
- Pulmonary capillary wedge pressure, mean: 14 mmHg (4-12 mmHg)
- Oxygen saturation: 40%

She was then started on antibiotics and pressors, and mixed etiology of shock was considered.

■ KEY POINTS

- Environmental and biomedical equipment play an important role in care of cardiac critical care unit (CCU) patients, and knowledge of these devices can guide the treatment in an efficient manner.
- Troubleshooting the equipment in CCU on a day-to-day basis is a challenging process and can improve patient outcomes.
- This chapter describes several devices used in the care of critically ill patients in the CCU.

■ NONINVASIVE BLOOD PRESSURE MEASUREMENT DEVICES

Introduction

Blood pressure measurements and goals should be based on the patient's risk of future complications and their previous cardiovascular history. Some indications for such patients are having atherosclerotic disease, heart failure, diabetes mellitus, or chronic kidney disease and being over 65 years old.

Patients who are admitted in the cardiac intensive care unit (ICU) after a cardiac arrest often have vasodilatory hypotension. It is suggested that a systolic blood pressure of 90 mmHg should be maintained with obtaining a mean arterial pressure (MAP) of 65 mmHg after a cardiac arrest. A systolic blood pressure less than 90 mmHg was associated with a higher mortality rate. Other studies supported a MAP goal of 65 to 80, which improved survival rate after arrest.

Mechanisms of Action

There are 2 ways to measure blood pressure:

- Oscillometric device (battery-operated device): This device involves sensing oscillations in pressure during the blood flow (Figure 12-1). The arterial flow to the limb is occluded by the pressure and then released gradually in order to sense the changes in blood flow. The faint blood flow correlates with the systolic pressure. Pulsatile oscillations increase to a maximum as pressure is released. This corresponds to the MAP and levels off at the level of the diastolic pressure.
- Sphygmomanometer (manual reading) in a situation in which an oscillometric reading cannot be obtained.

These 2 devices are used in the cases of noninvasive blood pressure monitoring.

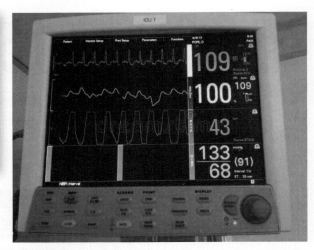

FIGURE 12-1. Bedside blood pressure monitor (oscilloscope). (See color insert.)

Cuff size and placement are equally important when attempting to get an accurate blood pressure measurement. Cuff bladder length should be about 80%, and width should be around 46% of upper arm circumference.

Indications

- It is vital to have blood pressure monitoring in the ICU setting to predict any future cardiac events or complications.
- An example of such a situation can be when the patient is being monitored when under anesthesia during and after a procedure. Circulatory system monitoring is crucial to prevent any complications with patients, especially in the ICU after surgery.
- Circulatory system monitoring can be done through clinical observation or by using physiologic monitors such as a blood pressure monitor.
- Blood pressure readings are crucial in case of a cardiovascular event. During surgery, blood pressure should be monitored every 5 minutes when the patient is under anesthesia and more frequently if needed based on the patient's clinical history and the type of procedure. If the procedure is invasive, then arterial blood pressure should also be monitored. Noninvasive blood pressure monitors are the standard devices used in the doctor's office. These are usually automatic.
- Blood pressure measurements and goals should be based on the patient's risk of future complications and previous cardiovascular history. Some indications for

such patients are having atherosclerotic disease, heart failure, diabetes mellitus, or chronic kidney disease or being older than 65.

Contraindications

- In some cases, regular automatic blood pressures may not be enough due to complicated cases. Other forms of vitals may be important for further evaluating the patient. Some of these vitals are the measurement of heart rate, electrocardiogram, and advanced cardiovascular monitors such as telemetry.[1]
- Patients with preexisting cardiovascular issues (diastolic pressure ≥110 mmHg) and patients older than 65 have supporting data for treatment and continuous blood pressure measurements to prevent future cardiovascular events and calculations. Good judgment calls should be made by physicians in these patients' cases as there is not enough data from other patient populations.

Complications

Accuracy of blood pressure measurement is crucial in predicting the cardiovascular health of a patient. There are multiple factors that can determine whether the reading will be accurate or not. These factors can lead to complications associated with inaccurate blood pressure readings. Although accuracy is usually excellent for noninvasive blood pressure, changes in blood pressure measurements that are either very low or extremely high are questionable.

- Higher measurements are usually seen generally in trauma patients with systolic blood pressure being less than 110 mmHg.
- Many of the measurement errors are related to the cuff size. Cuffs that are too large produce lower readings, whereas cuffs that are too small produce higher readings, leading to the inaccuracy
- Some other factors that give inaccurate blood pressure readings include patients who have issues with involuntary movements such as tremors and seizures. Other factors include severe hypotension, arrhythmias such as atrial fibrillation, and premature ventricular and atrial conductions.
- There can also be kinks and folds in the tubing or the cuff. Most importantly, repeated cuff inflations and blood pressures may lead to venous congestion that eventually leads to inaccurate blood pressure readings.[1]

- The positioning of the patient also plays a role in accurate blood pressure measurements. Hydrostatic changes can affect blood pressure measurements by increasing the readings. There can be an increase in "dependent" limbs and a decrease in the reading in elevated position of the limbs.

Troubleshooting

- Mistakes during blood pressure measurement can be corrected by properly positioning the patient. The 3 positions recommended are steep head up, steep head down, and sitting position.
- Positioning of the limbs is vital for accurate blood pressure measurements. Continuous blood pressure monitoring is recommended for patients with changes in blood pressure. Systolic and diastolic blood pressures are calculated, and certain devices are set according to manufacturer settings, meaning the accuracy depends on the algorithm used by the company.
- Oscillometric blood pressure devices have a time limit of 120 seconds to get a correct measurement. If the measurement is not obtained in this time frame, then a repeat blood pressure measurement is recommended.

■ BEDSIDE MONITORS

Introduction

Bedside monitors are screens used in a patient's room to monitor vital functions (Figure 12-2). They display heart rate, blood pressure, oxygen saturation, temperature, and

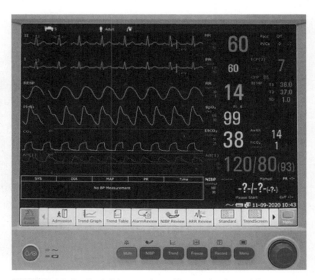

FIGURE 12-2. Bedside monitor. (See color insert.)

respiratory rate. Bedside monitors have multiple functions and can be used to display arterial line, central venous pressure (CVP), and PA catheter tracings.

Mechanism of Action

The monitor is connected with a wire and leads attached to the patient by stickers that have a sensing electrode. This sensor converts electrical signals to the waveform and displays it on the monitor. It has set parameters that can activate an alarm for clinician monitoring.

Indications

- All patients admitted in CCU are required to be on bedside monitors for detection of arrhythmia, hypoxia, or hypothermia/hyperthermia.
- It can display electrocardiogram and end-tidal carbon dioxide.
- Monitors are used for hemodynamic parameters display such as cardiac output, CVP, and PA pressures.
- It can show the trend of measurements for clinical record.

Contraindications

There are no contraindications, except if the patient or healthcare proxy refuses.

Equipment

Equipment includes monitor, cables, and connector with sensor.

Complications and Troubleshooting

- Error in interpretation and artifacts secondary to improper calibration, zeroing, or motion can occur that need clinical correlation.

■ HOSPITAL BEDS AND MATTRESSES

Mattresses are extremely important in a hospital setting, especially for patients who are going to be staying long term (Figure 12-3). Some of these patients are ICU and bariatric patients. Mattresses play an important role in preventing pressure-induced skin and soft tissue injury. Mattresses in the hospital are considered a type of support surface and hold an important role in pressure redistribution to provide injury protection during a patient's long-term stay, especially in the ICU. Mattresses also are important in prevention of chronic lower back pain. This can be a nonpharmacologic approach to improve the lives of patients who suffer from this condition.

Mechanisms of Action

Patients who are bedridden must have special attention given to proper positioning and repositioning every few hours even when the mattress is sufficient for care. This includes placement of pillows under legs and heels, positioning patients at an angle less than 30 degrees to prevent pressure exerted by bones, and elevation of the head

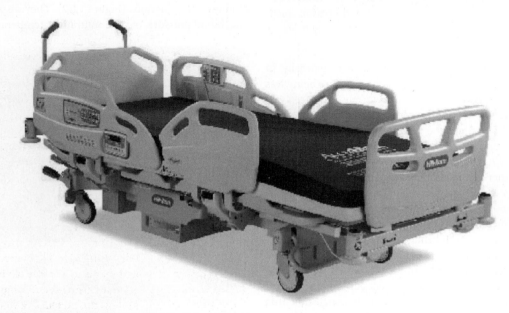

FIGURE 12-3. Hillrom CareAssist hospital bed.

less than 30 degrees to prevent any further injury related to friction. Multilayered foam dressings should be used when injuries and ulcerations cannot be prevented in predisposed patients.

Educating the staff and other individuals in direct care of patients is crucial in preventing pressure sores and maneuvering the mattress. Patient education documents should be at fifth-grade reading level and should be reviewed with the patient and family members.

Mechanical assistance is available for patients with severe obesity, such as inflatable lateral transfer mattresses. This is important for the staff and patient safety to prevent any injury related to weight.

Positioning of the patient should be checked regularly, especially for patients under anesthesia. Large patients may move when the bed is tilted. It is important that there is Velcro present between the bed and mattress in order to prevent slipping and falling of the patient.

Indications

- Low air loss mattresses should be chosen for patients who are obese. This will prevent the patients from sinking into the beds and will be more comfortable when they are trying to get out of bed. This is extremely important for preventing the breakdown of skin and sores that can develop over a long-term stay at the hospital.
- The mattresses should also be flexible in order for them to transform into a chair-like position so that the patients have easier access to the bathroom and other areas of the room.
- A mattress is directly placed on an existing surface, whether it is an ICU bed or an operating room table. There is evidence that highly specific foam mattresses used in the hospital bed and the mattresses used on operating tables reduce injury to patients receiving long-term care when compared to standard mattresses.
- There have also been many studies done that support the use of powered active air surfaces. These work a lot better at preventing injury than the standard hospital mattresses. Studies also support the use of powered mattresses over nonpowered mattresses. The powered mattresses redistribute the pressure in a timely manner so that tissue injury can be prevented.
- Specialized mattresses can be used for patients who suffer from chronic lower back pain. Lumbar supports and changes in sleeping surface may help reduce the incidence of painful episodes in such patients. Softer

mattresses that were back-conforming helped decrease pain and improve quality of life in patients with back pain compared to mattresses that were firm.

Contraindications

- Mattresses with high air loss may cause patients to sink, leading to the inability to get up and causing injuries. This may also lead to skin breakdown, ulcers, and injuries.
- Standard mattresses without toppers are not suggested for use by hospitals; instead, high-specification foam mattresses should be used.
- Patients who cannot stay in bed during their hospital stays are given full-seat cushions for the wheelchairs instead of donut cushions; donut cushions are not recommended due to an increase in edema and venous insufficiency.
- Even though powered mattresses are preferred, they are not cost effective compared to nonpowered mattresses. Given the high costs of powered mattresses, it is recommended to use support surfaces rather than a standard mattress in order to have similar benefits.
- Firm mattresses are contraindicated for patients living with chronic lower back pain. Several studies have supported the use of softer mattresses to improve the comfort level for these patients.

Complications

- Lack of provider and staff training may cause failure of preventive measures in reducing pressure-induced skin and soft tissue injury.
- Some patients are prone to getting these injuries because they are predisposed due to their medical conditions. Some of these conditions may include heart failure and terminal illnesses. Pressure-induced skin and soft tissue injuries are seen in the majority of the cases in the ICU. Nonpowered support surfaces such as foam mattresses should be used in combination with repositioning every 2 to 3 hours.
- Other complications include the potential spread of infection in mattresses. This is because some mattresses have an air circulation system, so airborne bacteria and spores can be absorbed by the pump. This can lead transfer of contaminants to a sterile environment. This is prevented in 2 ways: using filter pumps to filter out microbes and sealing the system. However, these solutions are not very cost-effective.

Troubleshooting

- Low air loss mattresses help support the patient's weight distribution. The mattresses are filled with deep cells, and these cells are ventilated. On these mattresses, the operating pressure can be set, and the mode of operation can be either static or cyclic. The cyclic mode can vary from mattress to mattress, and the internal air pressure changes. This helps with the redistribution of the load of the body weight over time.
- The air pressure is adjusted to an extent, depending on the load, and this is determined by the patient's body weight, shape, and position on the hospital bed.
- Each mattress should have an antimicrobial cover that does not create wrinkles. The wrinkles in the cover can lead to a pressure increase and tissue damage. The cover should also be waterproof to prevent bacterial growth.

■ AIR FILTRATION DEVICES AND HEPA FILTERS

Air filtration devices, such as high-efficiency particulate air (HEPA) filters, have been proposed in the healthcare setting to reduce the transmission of aerosolized infectious agents and allergens. They can be used in heating, ventilation, and air-conditioning systems in critical care units. The use of HEPA filters as a measure for infection control reduces the risk of infection and is recommended for patients at risk, such as those who are immunocompromised. Hospitals may choose from a number of manufacturers based on the filter's classification, ranging from H14 to H10, with H14 indicating an aerosol filtering efficiency of 99.9995% and H10 indicating an efficiency of 85% (H13 = 99.95%; H12 = 99.5%; H11 = 95%). Many studies have suggested less risk of fungal infection with filter use.

■ Mechanism of Action

The Centers for Disease Control and Prevention website defines a HEPA filter as a machine that can capture 0.3 μm of air particles with at least a 99.97% efficiency. The 0.3 μm is equivalent to the most penetrating particle size going through the filter. HEPA filters work by trapping and filtering small, harmful allergens and viruses/bacteria that may be airborne through a fine mesh.

Equipment

HEPA filters consist of the following:

- Outdoor air intake and exhaust duct
- Air handling unit
- Humidifier/compressor

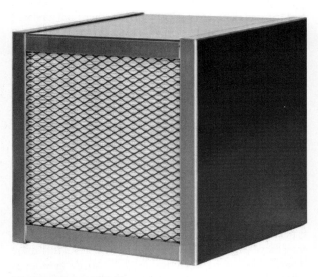

FIGURE 12-4. HEPA filter.

- Filters
- Noise attenuator

Indications

Whenever a HEPA filter is chosen, one has to weigh the risks versus benefits for each individualized patient.

- Patients who are particularly vulnerable to infections include those with deficient immune systems, chronic diseases such as diabetes mellitus, or cancer.
- Patients on immunosuppressive therapy such as chemotherapy also have an increased risk of infections.
- Other populations at risk include neonates, pregnant women, and those with concurrent infections, previous history of intubations, trauma, or certain surgical procedures, among others.

Contraindications

- Generally, contraindications include the presence of blood or any other thick secretions.
- Others include patients with pulmonary edema and those with an expired tidal volume of less than 70%.
- Filters should not be used in patients with a decreased tidal volume or those who are in acute respiratory failure.

Complications

Certain complications have been reported since the first use of HEPA filters, including tension pneumothorax due to positive-pressure air and pulmonary edema due to blockage of the filter presenting as hypoxia.

Troubleshooting

To troubleshoot, check the efficiency of the filter after a certain period. If the efficiency is below a certain point, it needs to be replaced.

■ INFUSION PUMPS

Introduction

According to the US Food and Drug Administration, an infusion pump is a device that allows a constant flow of nutrients and drugs into the patient. The user of an infusion pump can set the rate and duration of the feeding.

Mechanism of Action

An infusion pump is able to be customized to program the rate, duration, and dosage of the nutrients/drugs (Figure 12-5). Software then automatically releases the nutrients/drugs into the patient with the specifications that the technician set out.

Equipment

There are 2 types of infusion pumps:

- Traditional pump: In routine use for delivery of medication, fluids, and feedings.
- Specialty pump: Can be implantable, used for home care and for medication delivery such as insulin or pulmonary vasodilators (Figure 12-6).

Indications and Contraindications

- Pumps are used to deliver medication, fluids, or enteral/parenteral feeding at set rate and frequency.
- Patient-controlled pumps can be used to deliver analgesia in perioperative periods.
- Specialty pumps are used to deliver medication such as insulin and vasodilators after monitoring certain levels in blood.
- Pumps implanted in the body should be avoided if there is ongoing infection or coagulopathy or if the patient's comprehension is compromised.

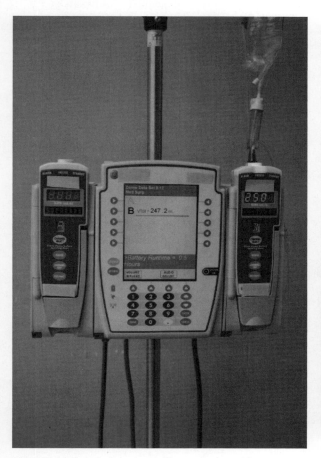

FIGURE 12-5. Infusion pump. (See color insert.)

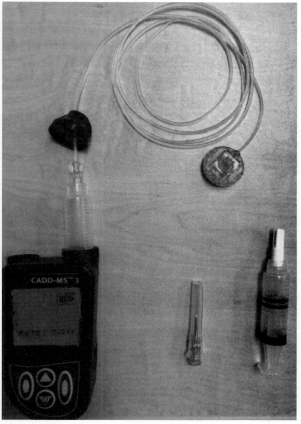

FIGURE 12-6. Remodulin subcutaneous pump. (See color insert.)

Complications

Complications may result from the simple fact that pumps are automatic, so devices may have to be checked every once in a while to make sure they are running smoothly. However, with the progression of automated technology, the newer infusion pumps are designed to alert if there is a problem such as a blockage in the tubing and even if the person may have an allergic reaction to the nutrient or drug.

Troubleshooting

- Infusion pump alarms can occur due to line occlusion, cord damage, or end of battery.

- To troubleshoot the infusion pump, the user has to verify the requirements that were laid out for each specific patient.
- The user may have to rest the machine manually to make sure the patient receives the correct specifications.

■ DEVICES USED IN CARDIAC CATHETERIZATION LABORATORY

In routine practice, the CCU receives patients from the catheterization laboratory. It is essential for a physician taking care of such patients to be familiar with certain equipment in the catheterization laboratory, which is described in Table 12-1.

■ TABLE 12-1. Procedures in the Catheterization Laboratory

Procedure	Indication	Access Site	Sheath Size	Anticoagulation Used	Antiplatelet Duration
Left heart catheterization	To assess LVEDP, and assess coronary angiogram	Radial or femoral artery	5-8 F	Heparin or bivalirudin (if PCI)	If PCI, DAPT for 6 months to 1 year
Right heart catheterization	Assess hemodynamics	Internal jugular, femoral, or antecubital vein	6-7 F	None	None
Pericardiocentesis	To remove fluids from pericardial space	Pericardial space	5 F	None	None
TAVR	Percutaneous aortic valve placement	Generally femoral artery, other options are transaortic or transapical	14-16 F	Heparin	DAPT for 6 months in general
Amplatzer PFO occluder	PFO closure	Femoral vein with atrial septal puncture	12-14 F	None	DAPT for 4-6 weeks
Watchman device	Left atrial appendage closure	Femoral vein with atrial septal puncture	12-14 F	No anticoagulation used but patient needs to be on it before procedure	Continue anticoagulation for 6 weeks

Abbreviations: DAPT, dual antiplatelet therapy; LVEDP, left ventricular end-diastolic pressure; PCI, percutaneous coronary intervention; PFO, patent foramen ovale; TAVR, transcatheter aortic valve replacement.

■ **TABLE 12-2. Vascular Closure Devices in the Catheterization Laboratory**

Device	Mechanism of Action	Site	Post Care
Perclose ProGlide	Suture delivery system	Femoral artery	Bedrest for 2 hours
Starclose	Nitinol clip	Femoral artery	Bedrest for 2 hours
Exoseal	Extravascular PGA plug	Femoral artery	Bedrest for 2 hours
Mynx	Extravascular PEG sealant	Femoral artery or vein	Bedrest for 2 hours
Vascade	Extravascular bioabsorbable closure	Femoral vein	Bedrest for 2 hours
Angioseal	Collagen plug at arteriotomy site	Femoral artery	Bedrest for 2 hours
TR band	Radial compression device	Radial artery	No bedrest, stays on wrist for 2 hours

Abbreviations: PEG, polyethylene glycol; PGA, polyglycolic acid; TR, tricuspid regurgitation.

■ VASCULAR CLOSURE DEVICES

See Table 12-2.

■ FUTURE DIRECTIONS

Physicians or clinical staff in the CCU will need in-service or refresher courses to familiarize themselves with procedures or devices used in other disciplines pertinent to patient care. Environmental and biomedical research is an area of ongoing interest in cardiac critical care.

SUGGESTED READINGS

Bartley JM, Olmsted RN, Haas J. Current views of health care design and construction: practical implications for safer, cleaner environments. *Am J Infect Control.* 2010;38:S1-12.

Curtis LT. Prevention of hospital-acquired infections: review of non-pharmacological interventions. *J Hosp Infect.* 2008;69:204-219.

Abbreviations

CCU: Cardiac critical care unit
CVP: Central venous pressure
ED: Emergency department
HEPA: High-efficiency particulate air
ICU: Intensive care unit
MAP: Mean arterial pressure
PA: Pulmonary artery

Index

Index

Index

Note: Page numbers followed by f indicate figures; those followed by t indicate tables.